O9-BUB-342

PRAISE FOR

THE EMPOWERED PATIENT

"Sharing her own personal struggles, CNN's Elizabeth Cohen gives keen insights on how you and your family can get excellent medical care from your doctor."

> —Deepak Chopra, author of *Reinventing the Body, Resurrecting the Soul*

"After generations of our treating health-care providers and doctors like gods, never questioning them and feeling complacent, Cohen's book is a wonderful shot in the arm. It's for all of us who want to approach medicine like consumers, to ask questions, and to know our rights. *The Empowered Patient* gives patients the valuable tools to advocate for themselves and their loved ones."

> —Lee Woodruff, author of *Perfectly Imperfect* and co-author with Bob Woodruff of *In an Instant*

"Just as our health-care system becomes more complex and each of us scrambles to find our place in the labyrinth, there is help. In *The Empowered Patient*, Elizabeth Cohen offers guidance for getting the most from your doctor, insurance company, and even your medicine. She outlines things you need to know when you are well, so that you have the voice and the power to access the system intelligently as a patient. This book will hold your hand, make you smart, and may even save your life."

> —Nancy L. Snyderman, MD, NBC News chief medical editor and author of *Diet Myths That Keep Us Fat*

"My colleague and friend Elizabeth Cohen has written a book no household should be without. With a no-nonsense approach to medicine, she will teach you how to do right by your bodies and your health care. One thing we all share in common is the likelihood that one day we will be a patient, and your best bet is to be an empowered patient. Let Elizabeth Cohen show you how."

> —Sanjay Gupta, MD, chief medical correspondent
> for the Health, Medical and Wellness unit at CNN
> and author of *Cheating Death*

"The minute I picked up *The Empowered Patient,* I knew this was a must-read book for everyone. Elizabeth Cohen reveals insider knowledge about the uncertainty of medicine—things every doctor knows—and then helps you steer a clear path to health!"

> —Christiane Northrup, MD, author of
> *Women's Bodies, Women's Wisdom* and
> *The Wisdom of Menopause*

"Whether you're seeking a second opinion, surfing the Internet for medical information, challenging doctors or nurses when treatments don't make sense, or confronting insurance denials or high pharmaceutical costs, CNN senior medical correspondent Elizabeth Cohen's provocative and saucy handbook is a gift. Her advice could be life-saving."

> —Bernadine Healy, MD, health editor and
> columnist, *U.S. News & World Report*

"It's not often one can say that reading a book will save your life. But Elizabeth Cohen's *The Empowered Patient* has the capacity to do just that. It's succinct, to the point, well organized, and packed with essential information for anyone facing hospital admission, meeting with a physician, or simply filling a prescription."

—Evan Handler, actor (*Sex and the City, Californication*), author of *Time on Fire* and *It's Only Temporary*, and long-term survivor of acute myeloid leukemia

"Elizabeth Cohen will teach you how to be your own best advocate for your health and your life. Elizabeth knows medicine inside-out as both an expert and as someone who almost died due to medical neglect. She has seen the best and the worst that medicine has to offer and will passionately guide you to empower yourself to get superior care for you or a loved one and save money at the same time." —Clark Howard, author of *Get Clark Smart*

THE
EMPOWERED
PATIENT

THE
EMPOWERED
PATIENT

How to Get the Right Diagnosis, Buy the Cheapest Drugs, Beat Your Insurance Company, and Get the Best Medical Care Every Time

ELIZABETH COHEN

BALLANTINE BOOKS TRADE PAPERBACKS

NEW YORK

As of press time, the URLs displayed in *The Empowered Patient* link or refer to existing websites on the Internet. Random House, Inc., is not responsible for, and should not be deemed to endorse or recommend, any website other than its own or any content available on the Internet (including without limitation any website, blog page, or information page) that is not created by Random House. The author, similarly, cannot be responsible for third-party material.

A Ballantine Books Trade Paperback Original

Copyright © 2010 by Elizabeth Cohen

All rights reserved.

Published in the United States by Ballantine Books, an imprint of The Random House Publishing Group, a division of Random House, Inc., New York.

BALLANTINE and colophon are registered trademarks of Random House, Inc.

LIBRARY OF CONGRESS CATALOGING-IN-PUBLICATION DATA
Cohen, Elizabeth.
The empowered patient: how to get the right diagnosis, buy the cheapest drugs, beat your insurance company, and get the best medical care every time / Elizabeth Cohen.
p. cm.
Includes bibliographical references and index.
ISBN 978-0-345-51374-8
1. Patient education. 2. Health counseling. I. Title.
R727.4.C64 2010
615.5071—dc22 2010019666

Printed in the United States of America

www.ballantinebooks.com

2 4 6 8 9 7 5 3 1

To Tal, who keeps his five gals healthy,
with all my heart

Contents

Introduction

Four days after giving birth, amped up on a combination of hormones and anxiety, I gathered together what was left of my stomach muscles and wrenched myself out of bed. Throwing on a bathrobe, I dragged myself to the neonatal intensive-care unit.

I'd been there before. Shir was our third daughter who had been in the NICU, and even at six-thirty in the morning, even in my postpartum fog, I knew the way through the winding corridors and up the elevator. From the looks of the men in the hallway, I probably had a breast or two hanging out of my robe, but I didn't care. That's how oblivious new mothers are to anything except their newborns. This holds especially true when that newborn is in intensive care, attached to IVs loaded with three antibiotics, two antiviral medications, and a monster dose of barbiturates.

When Shir was two days old, as I held her in my arms, she had a series of seizures that turned part of her face blue. The nurse whisked her upstairs from the maternity ward to the NICU, where neonatologists immediately put her on barbiturates, a standard treatment for seizures. Ever since, she'd been in a barbiturate-induced deep, deep sleep. She looked as if she were in a coma. For the next day and a half, we waited for a team of neurologists, cardiologists, hematologists, and infectious-disease experts to figure out the cause of her seizures. They feared it could be an infection, and so along with daily blood tests and urine tests she'd had a spinal tap every day, where doctors stuck a needle into her tiny spinal column to retrieve fluid. Not only is this procedure painful for the baby, it carries with it risks, such as infection, where the needle is inserted.

Finally, the night before my early-morning trip to the NICU, my husband and I received good news. The doctors had determined that the seizures were a fluke and weren't likely to happen again. They told us they would immediately stop the daily spinal taps, take her completely off the antibiotics and antivirals, and cut back on the massive doses of barbiturates that had made Shir so sleepy. In the morning we'd see a different baby, the doctors promised us, one who didn't have so many needles and was much more awake.

Relieved, my husband went home at midnight to be with our two older girls. On my early-morning jaunt to the NICU, I was filled with the hope of seeing my baby awake for the first time in two days.

That's not what I found.

When I arrived at the NICU that morning, Shir was the same rag doll I'd seen the night before; they hadn't decreased the barbiturates at all, and they hadn't taken her off the other medications. I asked the nurse on duty what was going on. Surely she'd received the doctors' orders the night before to stop the drugs and the spinal taps?

"There were no orders last night," she told me, checking the chart. "Everything's the same. They just gave her a spinal tap an hour ago."

What? They were supposed to stop the spinal taps immediately— our doctor had told us that for sure.

There was more. "That spinal tap they just gave her didn't work," the nurse told me. "They got the needle into her spine, and they tried but couldn't get any fluid out because she's dehydrated. They'll try again in an hour."

I couldn't believe what I was hearing. Not only had my baby had one unnecessary spinal tap; she was about to have another. I had to stop them.

"Call the doctor," I urged. "He'll tell you: she's not supposed to have any more spinal taps."

But the nurse refused. She repeated that Shir would have another spinal tap in an hour. No matter how much I argued, she was adamant.

Nothing had prepared me for this moment: the moment I would have to protect my daughter against a system bent on doing the wrong thing. Not my public-health degree, not my twelve years as a medical journalist at CNN, nothing. Every day I went on TV to explain medical news to the world. But even with that I couldn't stop this unnecessary, painful procedure from being performed unnecessarily—for the second time—on my tiny baby.

I decided that this wasn't going to happen. Not on my watch. I planted my sobbing self in a chair, blocking access to Shir's Isolette. When the doctor arrived to do the spinal tap, I would cut him off at the pass, reminding him that his colleagues had discontinued the spinal taps the night before.

"Oh no, you can't stay," the nurse came to tell me. "No visitors between seven and eight, when we change shifts," she said, pointing to a sign on the wall. "Come back at eight. They'll have done the spinal by then and you can discuss the results with the doctor."

She ushered me out of the NICU. Sobbing hard now, I felt that I had failed my daughter. No matter how much I begged the nurse, there seemed to be no way to prevent my baby from having a needle stuck into her spine for no reason whatsoever, and for the second time.

Back in my room, I cried so hysterically that I couldn't speak. Nurse after nurse came in to find out what was wrong, but I couldn't get even a syllable out. Finally, a nurse named Sarah managed to calm me down enough so that I could tell her what had happened.

"That's *bullshit*!" she said. "No way. I'm going right up there."

To this day, I have no idea what Sarah said, but within minutes I received a call from one of the neonatologists saying not to worry, there would be no more spinal taps, and they would start weaning Shir off the IV drugs. Finally, I had managed to protect my daughter. Through my tears, I had been an empowered patient.

When you go for your annual physical, your doctor will tell you to eat right and exercise, get tests like a mammogram or a colonoscopy, and take certain medications and vitamins to keep yourself healthy. That's great, but there are several important—vital, really—things your doctor doesn't tell you. He won't tell you, for example, that doctors often fail to communicate, with sometimes disastrous results, as I learned in the hospital with Shir. When your doctor admits you to the hospital, he won't tell you how truly dangerous a place a hospital really is. Some 99,000 Americans die each year from infections they acquire in the hospital, and as many as another 98,000 die from medical mistakes in the hospital. Taken together, these hospital dangers kill more people than breast cancer, prostate cancer, car accidents, AIDS, and diabetes *combined*.

Your doctor won't alert you to these dangers, but I will. And there's more. You don't have to be in the hospital to fall victim to the shortcomings of our health-care system; you just have to go to see the doctor. Studies tell us that when you go to the doctor with a health problem his diagnosis will be wrong as many as one out of every four times. If you have a lump and the doctor does a biopsy and sends the specimen to a lab to see if it's cancer, more than one time out of ten the pathologist in the lab will make the wrong call. When the test results come back to your doctor's office, there's a good chance the doctor will never call and give you the results—even when the results are bad news and you need treatment fast.

I'm sure that at your next appointment your doctor won't tell you this: physicians play favorites. Women are less likely than men to get the right treatment for a heart attack and many other medical ailments. African-Americans are less likely to get expensive lifesaving treatments even when they have the same medical insurance as white people. Studies have shown that doctors are less likely to spend time with overweight patients. Here's something else your doctor won't tell you about himself: he almost surely has relationships with pharmaceutical companies that influence the choice of drugs he prescribes for you.

Since your doctor won't tell you these things, I will. I'll also tell you what to do about them. I'll tell you how to keep a hospital from killing you, and what steps you need to take to ensure that you get the right diagnosis. And did you know that if you've been waiting in the ER for a long time you can pick up a house phone and ask for the administrator on call? Or that if the price tag for your prescription drug is through the roof your pharmacist can ask your physician to suggest a less expensive drug that will work just as well? Did you know that using certain key words in a letter to your health-insurance company will make it much more likely to pay for an expensive procedure?

Along the way, I'll introduce you to my patient heroes, people who knew more than their doctors did and bucked the system in order to get the care they needed. There's Suzanne, who practically threw herself on the hospital bed when a nurse refused to give her daughter an anesthetic before a painful procedure. There's Albert, who had to step in and stop a nurse from giving his wife a double dose of a medication. There's Jessica, a high school senior, who diagnosed her own Crohn's disease in her science class. There's my sister, Julia, who had to play detective to find a fertility treatment when her doctor refused to lay out all her options. Then there's the actor Dennis Quaid, who became a patient-safety activist after his newborn twin babies received an enormous drug overdose in the hospital that nearly killed them.

I'm writing this book so that you, too, won't have to suffer. Never in the history of modern American health care has there been such an urgent and dramatic need to advocate for yourself and the people you love at the doctor's office and in the hospital. But here's the good news: you can do it. You're in control. Just as Suze Orman taught so many of us to take control of our finances, I can teach you how to do the same for your medical care. You *do* have the power to get the best medical care for you and the people you love. In this book, I'll answer these questions for you:

- How do I make sure a hospital doesn't kill me with a medication error or infection?
- How do I know if a doctor has misdiagnosed my condition?
- How do I make sure I have the best doctor?
- How do I get the most out of the short time I have with my doctor?

I want to be clear: I'm not one of those people who believes health care in the United States is a complete disaster. Despite what Michael Moore says, the United States has some of the best care in the world, and my family and I have been grateful recipients of it on many occasions. But getting that excellent care takes know-how, and I want to share with you what I've learned through my reporting and my personal experiences with doctors. In my book, you'll learn the health-care mistakes that are most likely to kill you, and what you can do to keep from becoming a victim.

Remember, doctors are smart, but they don't know everything. You have to take charge.

This isn't a book about complaining. I'll tell you what your doctor doesn't so you can get the best medical care possible. Your life, or the life of someone you love, may depend on it.

THE
EMPOWERED
PATIENT

CHAPTER ONE

How to Be a "Bad Patient"

You probably know Evan Handler as Harry Goldenblatt, Charlotte York's adorable, bald husband on *Sex and the City,* or as Charlie Runkle, the agent for David Duchovny's character on *Californication.* What you probably don't know is that Evan Handler was a "bad patient"—a patient so bad doctors dreaded him and nurses cursed him. But Handler swears that being a bad patient saved his life.

When Handler was diagnosed with leukemia at the age of twenty-three, his doctors told him he probably wouldn't survive, and so Handler eventually left those doctors and found others across the country who were more optimistic. When Handler was undergoing chemotherapy, a doctor yelled at him for calling about a fever because the fever was "only" 100 degrees. Handler fired him. "Doctors told me I would be endangering my care if I switched doctors, but that advice was criminal," he told me. He continued this "bad patient" behavior even after he recovered from cancer. "Recently I needed to have something in my mouth looked at," Handler told me. "The doctor performed a biopsy without lidocaine—just put a blade in my mouth and cut without telling me. I never went back, and I wrote him a three-page letter. You should leave a bad doctor and, if you have the energy, tell him why you left."

Several times in the hospital when he was in his twenties, nurses tried to give Handler a medication that his doctor had absolutely forbidden, and he had to argue with the nurses each time to stop them from administering the dangerous drug. Once, a nurse gave him an intravenous medicine that was meant for another patient—the other patient's name was right there on the bag—and Handler was the one to notice the mistake. When hospital workers didn't wear gloves and gowns—the proper procedure when taking care of patients whose immune system has been zapped into nothingness—he told them to suit up. When doctors told Handler it would take days to replace an infected catheter, he fought for it to be done right away.

Handler took being a "bad patient" to new levels. For example, he became exasperated when one lab took a long time to process blood tests, delaying his physician's ability to prescribe the right treatments, and so he found a different lab that did the job more expeditiously. The doctor's orders, however, were for the first lab, not the second, so Handler became what he described as "a criminal of sorts" by forging his doctor's signature on authorization slips. I asked him if he was afraid he'd get caught. "Nothing bad is going to happen to you if you don't do exactly as you're told," he answered. "They weren't going to put me in jail. I worried about getting caught only because then I wouldn't be able to do it anymore."

Handler says that he survived cancer, ten hospitalizations, multiple rounds of chemotherapy, and one life-threatening infection after another by being a "bad patient." "The irony of being a 'bad' patient is that they actually do better for themselves than 'good patients,' " he told me. In his book *Time on Fire* he wrote, "I learned that I must always remain in control, double-check everyone's work, and trust no one completely. I must have been sheer hell to be around. But I know that my cantankerousness saved my life on several occasions." When he was too sick to fight for himself, his girlfriend stepped in. "I was his protector for much of the time in the hospital," Jackie Reingold, his former girlfriend, told *The New York Times*. "We stood up for our rights and our dignity. So we were yelled at a lot by nurses." Handler says he knows some people aren't lucky enough to have an advocate by their side. "You wonder how many people die from illnesses because their strength to keep up vigilance runs out?"

As the senior medical correspondent for CNN, every week since July 2007 I've written a column for cnn.com called "Empowered Patient." In my column I write about people like Evan Handler—people who have struggled with misdiagnoses and rushed doctors, with insurance companies that refuse to pay up, with medication mistakes and medical neglect. When I first started the column, I wasn't sure stories like Evan Handler's would resonate with the general public. After all, most people, thank goodness, never get a horrible disease like cancer, so they never get a chance (thank goodness again) to experience the shortfalls of our current medical system. But week after week I've proved myself wrong. The comments in the Sound Off sections under my weekly articles clearly show that Americans are mad as hell about their health care. "I barely get to see my doctor, and when I do I wait two hours for ten minutes of rapid discussion about my health," one reader wrote. "My HEALTH. I spend more time with my auto mechanic." From another: "I can't think of any other profession where the ones paying for the services are treated with so little respect." A third wrote, "The doctor gave us 22 seconds (I timed it) of his time and dismissed us."

Many readers have recounted horror stories about doctors who missed their cancer, pharmacies that gave them someone else's prescription, medical records that were confused with someone else's, surgeons who nearly operated on the wrong side of the body, and even a surgeon who performed an operation that was meant for someone else. (The patient realized the mistake when a nurse called him by the wrong name.) Readers were quite direct about their dissatisfaction. "Doctors need to get over themselves," "Doctors don't care and are a waste of money," "Doctors think they are gods," and "Doctors are generally idiots" are just some of the comments I've received.

Often readers resort to sarcasm, as in this comment to doctors: "Awww, your malpractice insurance is SO high? I bet you cry all the way home in your Mercedes to your $300,000 home." I'm sure some of these readers are just malcontents, but if even a fraction of these patients are describing real situations and real misdiagnoses and real medical errors there's something very seriously wrong with our system, because it's a system where you lose if you're good.

You Know You're a "Good Patient" When . . .

1. You worry about what your doctor thinks of you.
2. You worry about insulting your doctor.
3. You worry about sounding stupid in front of your doctor.
4. You think repeatedly about leaving your doctor and finding a new one, but you don't.
5. You're too scared to tell your doctor you'd like to get a second opinion.
6. You stick with a doctor who's been treating you for a long time for the same problem, and you're not getting better. If you took your car to the mechanic repeatedly and the car was still broken, would you stay with that mechanic?
7. When you don't get satisfying answers to your questions, you stop asking.

BARBARA AND STEPHANIE: THE DANGER OF BEING A "GOOD PATIENT"

Being a "bad patient" is crucial to mastering the skills I teach in this book. Many of us (and I include myself in this group) have a very hard time being bad. It involves exercising a certain level of mistrust we don't usually exercise in our regular lives. (Even the president of the United States, a savvy man, presumably, has indicated an unquestioning trust in doctors. "The fact is Americans, and I include myself and Michelle and our kids in this, we just do what you tell us to do," Barack Obama told a gathering of the members of the American Medical Association in 2009. "That's what we do. We listen to you. We trust you.") Being a "bad patient" also involves a level of aggressiveness—openly questioning doctors, being in-your-face with nurses—that's pretty foreign to me; it's just not the way I operate. After interviewing hundreds of patients over the years, I've discovered that many people feel this way.

That's why I wish I could have introduced Evan Handler to Barbara Robbins ten years ago. Barbara could have used a dose of Handler's bad-patient-ness when her daughter Stephanie turned thirteen and started losing weight dramatically. Every time Stephanie ate, she had cramps and bloody diarrhea. Consuming just a morsel of food sent her running to the bathroom; the need came urgently and without warning. To avoid the pain, not to mention the embarrassment, Stephanie ate as little as possible. Barbara took Stephanie to a gastroenterologist, who diagnosed irritable bowel syndrome, and for the next eight years Stephanie tried one drug after another. Some worked better than others, but still, by the time she reached high school Stephanie's weight had dipped to 113 pounds—and she's six feet tall. Her illness ruled her life. She couldn't attend events like high school football games, because the bathroom was too far away from the stands. She even left a college she loved because to go there she had to take the elevated train that runs through Chicago and there were no toilets. But through all this, Barbara never questioned the doctor's diagnosis or treatment plan. "I figured he knew best," she said. "Up until that point, I'd only had good experiences with doctors, so I had no reason to doubt his judgment. I figured the doctor must know more than I did."

In the end, a crisis finally opened Barbara's eyes. When Stephanie was around twenty-three, the gastroenterologist prescribed yet another new drug for her cramps and diarrhea. Stephanie very quickly spiked a high fever and in six hours had twenty-six bloody bowel movements. Barbara rushed her daughter to the hospital, where the gastroenterologist immediately took Stephanie off the new drug. Stephanie's fever went down, and the bloody diarrhea stopped. Barbara was relieved. Then the doctor did a curious thing. He put Stephanie back on the drug, and the fever and diarrhea returned. When Barbara asked why he'd done that, the gastroenterologist asserted that the drug couldn't possibly be causing the problems, since the medical literature contained no reports that this drug had those particular side effects.

Barbara was dumbfounded. She was no doctor, but she knew what she was seeing with her own eyes. On the drug her daughter was extremely ill, and off the drug she was better. Back on the drug, the symptoms returned. Yet the doctor refused to admit that a drug he'd prescribed could be making Stephanie sick. At first, Barbara didn't say anything. "It was like my tongue was bolted to the bottom of my mouth, and I couldn't get the words out," she told me. "I didn't want to offend him. I was paralyzed." But then something struck her. "Right there, at that very moment in my daughter's hospital room, it hit me that this doctor was wrong, and that there was a good chance he'd been wrong from the very beginning," Barbara recalled. "I told him I was taking Stephanie to the University of Chicago to get a second opinion. He had a cow. He was so angry he was shaking. He said I was overreacting and he hadn't finished going through all the different drug regimens yet, that there were still more drugs to try. I said, 'We've been trying these drugs for ten years and they're not working. Do you expect my daughter to continue to suffer?' That's when he walked out."

Four years later, Barbara can still remember the sound of the door slamming behind the doctor as he stormed out of her daughter's hospital room. From that moment on—from the moment she learned not to trust doctors implicitly—everything fell into place. The surgeon at the University of Chicago said that Stephanie had never had IBS; she actually had ulcerative colitis, an inflammation of the lining of the large intestine and the rectum. Other doctors agreed with his diagnosis, and so the surgeon removed her colon, which is sometimes done in severe cases of ulcerative colitis. Once she recovered from complications of the surgery, she gained five pounds in one month. Today she weighs 160 pounds, a healthy weight for her six-foot frame. Stephanie suffered needlessly for ten years. It didn't have to happen. If her mother had been a "bad patient," she could have been treated successfully at thirteen instead of twenty-three.

WHAT THE STUDIES SAY

You go to the doctor's office for a test. You're told that the doctor will get back to you in a few days with the results, but a week later you haven't heard anything. If you're a "good patient," you assume the doctor knows what she's doing and everything's fine. This would be a very dangerous assumption to make. A 2009 study by doctors at Weill Cornell Medical College in New York found that more than 7 percent of the time doctors failed to inform patients when they've had an abnormal test result. This means that for every fourteen abnormal tests you have, your doctor's office will fail to inform you about results for one of them. We're not talking about minor tests, but about tests like mammograms and colonoscopies, which can save your life.

A "bad patient" wins in this situation, because she badgers the doctor's office for results instead of figuring that no news is good news. Here's another case where the "bad patient" wins: when discharging a patient from the hospital, doctors and nurses, who are often in a rush these days, sometimes fail to give patients complete instructions on how to care for themselves at home. If you're a "good patient," you nod your head and don't ask too many questions because you pick up on the doctor's or nurse's body language that he wants to hightail it over to the next patient. The "bad patient" keeps asking questions until she understands absolutely everything, even if the doctor or the nurse is visibly annoyed. The payoff for doing this is big: a study published by the Agency for Healthcare Research and Quality found that patients who clearly understood their discharge instructions were 30 percent less likely to be readmitted to the hospital or visit the emergency department. Being a "bad patient" can keep you from winding up back in the hospital.

Why You Need to Be a Bad Girl

Please forgive me a gross generalization here: I think women have an especially hard time being "bad patients." I think too many of us want to be good girls in every situation, including at the doctor's office. Dr. Christiane Northrup, the author of *Women's Bodies, Women's Wisdom: Creating Physical and Emotional Health and Healing,* agrees. "There are literally hundreds of situations in which a woman's gut intuition is spot-on, but she talks herself out of it so as not to make waves," Northrup tells me. "We women are suckers for wanting to be loved." As we saw with Barbara, who overly trusted her daughter's doctor, it doesn't matter how many degrees you have. "Even very well-educated women sometimes freeze up and don't speak up," Northrup says.

If you think you're that good girl, then it's especially important that you not go it alone. "Always take someone with you who will ask the questions you are afraid to ask," Northrup advises.

SOLUTION: HOW TO BE A SUCCESSFUL "BAD PATIENT"

I think Dr. Andrew Weil, bestselling author and founder of the Arizona Center for Integrative Medicine, put it beautifully when he told me, "Disempowerment adds to a patient's distress and is an obstacle to recovery. Do not be passive. Remember, it is the 'difficult' patients who often have the best outcomes." But what do you do if you're like me (or, apparently, Barack Obama) and your instincts tell you to trust your doctor? If you're naturally a "good patient," it won't be easy to switch that off and become a "bad patient." Luckily, it is possible to be a bad patient without becoming an obnoxious one.

Let's use Barbara as an example. She had a dilemma: her daughter Stephanie wasn't getting better after years in her doctor's care. If Barbara had channeled her inner Evan Handler and been skeptical about the doctor's diagnosis, she could have said to the doctor, "We've been seeing you for this problem for a year, and none of the treatments we've tried have worked. Do we need to rethink our approach, or should we consider seeing another physician?" Here's another "good-patient dilemma" and "bad-patient solution." Let's say your doctor's staff is terrible about calling you back with test results. The "bad-patient solution" is to face this head-on, saying something like "It took your office two weeks to get back to me about a lab test. I know your office is busy, but that's a long time. Any thoughts on how we could do things more quickly?" The ultimate "good-patient dilemma" is that you worry about what your doctor thinks of you. The solution to this one is easy: remember that your relationship with your doctor is a business relationship (after all, that's really what it is). You pay her, and she takes care of your medical problems. End of story.

Now that we know how to solve these good-patient dilemmas, let's think about why it took Barbara ten years and a near-catastrophe to finally start questioning her doctor. After all, she's one tough lady: she raised Stephanie and Stephanie's sister by herself after her husband died, she has a PhD, and she's the dean of a graduate school at a major university. At work, she has to disagree with people all the time, stand up for herself, and make decisions that sometimes make people mad. Why couldn't she do that in the doctor's office?

I asked Dr. Jerome Groopman, the author of the brilliant book *How Doctors Think,* for his thoughts on the question, and he told me how he was willing to let a surgeon go in and operate on his painful wrist even though the surgeon had no idea what was wrong or what he would do once he got in there. "Why did you trust that doctor when, really, his plan sounded pretty stupid?" I asked Dr. Groopman. He thought about it for a minute. "Look. You're sick. You're desperate. You're like a child and the doctor is the parent," he told me. "Like a little child, we want to trust the parent who can get us out of danger." Also, most of us just naturally hate confrontation with anyone. Dr. Groopman remembers, for example, when he felt that his internist was becoming too busy to give him good care at a time when he needed him most, but he didn't want to confront him. "It sounds strange, but I didn't want to insult him," he said.

I've spoken to other doctors who have noticed that, despite all their knowledge and training, they don't think clearly and critically about health care when they're the patient. One patient advocate, Dr. Michael Victoroff, calls it "the fog of the examining room." "I have a friend who has an MD and an MBA, and he says when he's the patient the minute he walks into the examining room his IQ goes down thirty points," Dr. Victoroff told me.

If doctors can get lost in the fog, it's no wonder Barbara got lost. But just remember the huge payoff for being a "bad patient." As we saw with Evan Handler, being a "bad patient" saved his life, and as we saw with Barbara, being a "good patient" caused her daughter ten years of needless suffering. Thankfully, Stephanie is in good health today. She's twenty-seven and in nursing school, hoping to treat patients better than she was treated. I asked her if she thought things had changed, if young people like her were better at being their own advocates compared with her mother and others in the Marcus Welby generation. "You know what—I really don't think so," she said. "Even people in my class at nursing school, who should know better, blindly trust that the doctor is always right. Really, in the end it's all about having as much say in your care as the doctor does."

Final Checklist: The Three Golden Rules of Being a "Bad Patient"

1. **Ask lots of questions.** If you don't understand something, ask for clarification, and if you still don't understand, ask again. The doctor or nurse might be visibly annoyed, but that shouldn't stop you. Remember, your health depends on your ability to comprehend what the doctor is telling you.

2. **Don't worry whether your doctor likes you.** If you worry whether your doctor likes you, you could be putting your health in jeopardy, because you'll be hesitant to do anything that might upset the doctor, such as asking lots of questions. Remember that while it's a natural inclination to want to be liked, your health comes first and your popularity second.

3. **Remember that this is a business transaction.** You're paying the doctor for a service, just as you would pay a car mechanic or the person who cleans your house. Of course, you're respectful of your doctor, just as you're respectful of the mechanic or the housekeeper, but you don't owe it to your doctor to be the perfect patient.

CHAPTER TWO

How to Find Dr. Right
(and Fire Dr. Wrong)

Did you ever see the *Seinfeld* episode where Elaine gets into trouble at the doctor's office? While she's waiting in the examining room, she sneaks a peek at her chart and notices that it says she's "difficult." When the doctor comes in, he whips the chart out of her hands.

DOCTOR: You shouldn't be reading that.

ELAINE: Well, it's, you know, I noticed that somebody wrote in my chart that I was difficult in January of '92, and I have to tell you that I remember that appointment exactly. You see, this nurse asked me to put a gown on, but it was a mole on my shoulder and I specifically wore a tank top so I wouldn't have to put a gown on. You know, they're made of . . . paper.

DOCTOR: Well, that was a long time ago. How about if I just erase it. Now, about that rash—

ELAINE: But it was pen. You fake-erased.

(Annoyed with Elaine, the doctor makes a beeline for the door.)

DOCTOR *(on his way out the door)*: "This doesn't look too serious. You'll be fine."

Screenwriter Jennifer Crittenden told me that she wrote this *Seinfeld* script because she'd had a "difficult patient" moment of her own in real life. One day she arrived for her dermatologist appointment on time but ended up sitting in the examining room, drumming her fingers, waiting for the doctor to show up. She looked up at the clock, realized she was about to be very late for work, took off the paper gown, got dressed, walked out of the examining room, and rescheduled with the receptionist. When she returned for the new appointment, she again had a long wait in the examining room. This time, like Elaine, Crittenden peeked at her chart. She found that the receptionist had written she'd been "very angry" at the last appointment. "I felt like it was an odd thing to put in a medical chart, not to mention an unfair characterization of the incident," Crittenden told me. She fired the dermatologist and found herself a new one.

Go, Jennifer! We all deserve Dr. Right. Having Dr. Right might not seem very important if you're healthy, but when you're sick having Dr. Right could save your life. Dr. Right will call you back when you have a question about your medications. Dr. Right will act on a test result instead of letting it sit on his desk for weeks. If you're in the emergency room and no one's paying attention to you, Dr. Right will call the triage nurses and light a fire under them. Dr. Right isn't just chosen at random from your insurance company's list of physicians. Dr. Right is someone who comes recommended by someone you know and trust. Dr. Right has experience dealing with your particular medical problem. Dr. Right hasn't been blasted repeatedly on doctor-rating websites. Dr. Right is someone who hasn't been censured by her state licensing board. And, perhaps above all, *Dr. Right is someone you like and who likes you.*

FIXING MY MOTHER UP WITH DR. RIGHT

My mother has end-stage kidney failure, which means that she needs a new kidney. While she waits for one—and it could be years before she gets one, if ever—Mom will have to go on dialysis, where she'll be tethered to a machine six days a week to clean out the toxins that her withering kidneys can no longer filter.

The worst part of all this is that it wasn't inevitable. My mother might be healthy today if only she'd found Dr. Right.

Mom has always enjoyed pretty good health, but when she was sixty, she began to feel tired, achy, and dizzy. She went to the doctor, and he noticed that along with these symptoms her blood pressure was borderline high, despite the fact that she was on blood-pressure medication. Her internist tinkered with different medications and dosages, but the achiness didn't go away, and her blood pressure wouldn't budge. The internist then proceeded to tell my mother that her blood pressure would go down if she just stopped working so hard. "He told me the high blood pressure and the other problems came from being so busy. Slow down, he said, and you'll be okay," my mother recalls.

This response sounded strange to me. My mother had worked hard—and had done so happily—all her adult life, and until now she'd felt fine. Why all of a sudden would her long days (she's a lawyer, social worker, and grandmother) cause her to feel ill?

My mother's health continued to deteriorate. While visiting me in Atlanta, she felt especially weak, so I took her to my internist. He listened to her history, noting the tinkering with the medications, and sat and thought for a good long while. When you get back home, he told her, ask your doctor to check out your adrenal glands. Tiny things that sit atop your kidneys, adrenal glands play a major role in regulating blood pressure. When my mother returned home, she saw a new internist, who immediately sent her to a nephrologist, a doctor who specializes in the kidneys. He did several blood tests, which indicated that her kidneys were out of whack. Based on these test results, the nephrologist ordered more tests, confirming an adrenal abnormality.

If my mother's original internist had caught her adrenal problem earlier, in all likelihood surgery could have corrected it. But at this stage, surgery wasn't an option. Her nephrologist could treat her only with medicines and changes in her diet. This doctor did a great job, and my mother did exactly as she was told, but ten years after her diagnosis the day we all feared arrived. The doctor informed her that the medicines and the dietary changes were no longer working: she was in end-stage kidney failure. Only a kidney transplant or dialysis would keep her alive.

If the original internist had ordered a simple blood test instead of blaming my mother's symptoms on her work, she probably wouldn't be in the situation she's in now. So why *hadn't* the doctor ordered a few simple blood tests when he saw that my mother's blood pressure all of a sudden wasn't responding to medication, and when, out of nowhere, she started to feel tired and achy? Why did he blame *her* for her rising blood pressure? I can't help wondering: if she'd been a sixty-year-old male CEO, would he so glibly have dismissed her problem as one of simply "working too hard"? Would he have patted a man on the head and told him to relax? Or would he have done more tests to get at the root of the problem?

If there's one thing you should take away from this book it's that *you must find a doctor who takes you and your health problems seriously.* Dr. Right won't attribute your problems to being "all in your head." Dr. Right won't tell you that if you "just relax" your symptoms will go away. If my mother had found Dr. Right from the very beginning, things probably would have turned out very differently. The lesson to learn from my mother's experience is that a doctor who blames you for your illness is Dr. Wrong. Finding Dr. Right could have saved my mother's kidneys.

Finding Dr. Right Can Save Your Life

Erica Gero says she owes her life to Doreen Kossove, who convinced her—badgered her, really—into finding Dr. Right.

Gero met Dr. Kossove on the website for the Association of Cancer Online Resources. The two women were fighting the same rare cancer called leiomyosarcoma, and Dr. Kossove, a pediatrician, advised patients like Gero from a laptop in her sickbed, doling out advice even as she herself lay dying. She told Gero to ditch her doctor and find one who had experience treating their particular type of cancer. Gero says Dr. Kossove's insistence made her switch doctors, and that the new doctor gave her the treatment that saved her life. "Doreen gritted her teeth and would not let go of me until I went to the right kind of doctor," Gero wrote on ACOR's website. "She was polite, but snarky at the same time. And of course she was right. I owe her my life." Gero wasn't the only cancer patient Dr. Kossove counseled, and she did it voluntarily. "[I have] about 2,000 rare-cancer patients under my gimlet stare," Kossove wrote about the patients she helped online. Sometimes she showed impatience when people on the site stayed too long with the wrong doctor. "I get very exasperated, very bitter and very worried about the people on this list," she wrote to one woman. "[Some of them] put their heads in the sand."

With a mother-hen style, Dr. Kossove pushed the cancer patients under her "gimlet stare" to hire the right doctor, fire the wrong doctor, and find the latest treatments, which can be very difficult for rare cancers. She urged them to question doctors who told them there were no options left. In 2001, doctors told Dr. Kossove that she had only a month to live. She died in 2009 at the age of sixty-five, having helped legions of grateful cancer patients live longer and healthier lives.

WHAT THE STUDIES SAY

In his landmark book *Blink,* Malcolm Gladwell describes how when we meet people for the first time we reach conclusions about them in the blink of an eye. It's not conscious, but we all make judgments about people based on all sorts of things, such as how they're dressed or what they look like. Doctors, being human beings, also do this. Some physicians, like Dr. Jennifer Griggs, an oncologist and an associate professor at the University of Michigan Medical School, recognize this, and try to explain to other doctors that without even knowing it they have preconceived notions about their patients. "When I give speeches, I ask doctors to close their eyes and picture a librarian," she says. "Everyone pictures the same person—the one with the bun in her hair who's always saying 'Shh' and probably goes home and curls up with her cat and a good book after work." Dr. Griggs is right: there may very well be librarians out there with purple hair and nose rings who spend their weekends headbanging in mosh pits, but that's not the librarian we all picture.

So what does this mosh pit–loving librarian have to do with finding Dr. Right? Everything. You want to find a doctor whose "blink" assessment of you is right-on and positive. If you think doctors don't harbor negative thoughts about patients, you should think again. In fact, the phenomenon of doctors disliking patients is so widespread that physicians have developed a rich vocabulary for the patients they find distasteful. "Turkeys," "trolls," "crocks," and "GOMERS" (for "Get out of my emergency room") are just a few of the names doctors have for patients they don't like. "Heartsink" patients make the doctor's heart sink every time their name appears on the daily schedule. Patients who come in with a stack of Internet printouts are called "brainsuckers." In all, studies show that doctors consider up to 30 percent of their patients to be difficult. So the next time you're in the waiting room, look to your left and look to your right, and odds are one of you will be deemed "difficult" by the doctor you're waiting to see.

If your doctor thinks you're difficult, this is more than just a personality clash: it will affect your health. Do you think a doctor who finds you difficult will give you excellent care? No way. A physician who considers you a "brainsucker" won't thoroughly think through your diagnosis. One who regards you as a royal pain in the neck won't take the time to carefully review all your treatment options.

Clearly, a doctor who thinks you're difficult isn't Dr. Right. A few honest physicians have spoken openly about their dislike of certain patients—and how this attitude damages the care they give these patients. In an article titled "Torment," Dr. Danielle Ofri, an assistant professor of medicine at New York University School of Medicine, wrote, "I groan when I catch sight of her name on the patient roster." Whenever she sees "Mrs. Uddin," Dr. Ofri experiences "a dull cringing in my stomach that gradually creeps outward, until my entire body is sapped by foreboding and dread. . . . I start to resent her, to hate her, to hate everything about her." Dr. Ofri can't stand hearing about Mrs. Uddin's problems. "There is abdominal pain and headache, diarrhea and insomnia, back pain and aching feet, a rash and gas pains, itchy ears and a cough, no appetite. And more headache . . . I begin to ignore a certain percentage of what is being said. . . . I stop believing what she tells me are her symptoms. . . . Stop it, I want to yell at her. Just stop complaining. Go away. Stop bothering me." The important part here is that because Dr. Ofri dislikes Mrs. Uddin so intensely she stops giving Mrs. Uddin the proper care, since it's tough to treat a patient effectively when you're no longer listening to her. In the end, with the help of Mrs. Uddin's daughter, Dr. Ofri comes to understand her patient's problems and gets her the help she needs.

Dr. Wendy Levinson, chair of the American Board of Internal Medicine and chair of the Department of Medicine at the University of Toronto, once wrote about a patient she dreaded. "Mary" reached Dr. Levinson through the answering service late at night and on weekends, "always complaining of increased [back] pain I felt helpless to correct. . . . She was forever angry with me." At every appointment, Mary insisted on narcotics for her pain, and Dr. Levinson refused them. "I hated this patient. I just could not stand her," Dr. Levinson told me. Like Dr. Ofri with Mrs. Uddin, Dr. Levinson came to realize that she was so annoyed by Mary that she couldn't truly help her. "I just wasn't giving her the right treatment," she explained.

Discouraged, Dr. Levinson sought the advice of a psychologist friend, who suggested a technique called "mining for gold," which means looking for something—anything—to like about a tiresome person. She took her friend's advice, and realized she didn't know much about Mary's children, who were ages six and eight. When she asked about them, Mary grew excited talking about her older daughter's achievements in track and field. "I have three young children myself and somehow Mary and I shared a bond of caring and commitment to our kids," Dr. Levinson wrote. "Mary was delighted that I seemed so interested in learning more about her children and I think she started to feel like I was genuinely concerned about her." As time went on, Mary was willing to take Dr. Levinson's suggestions to try physical therapy, injections in her back, and pills that weren't narcotics. Mary complained less and stopped calling Dr. Levinson as often at night and on weekends. As Dr. Levinson explained to me, when she hated Mary she found herself delivering substandard care. When she found something to like about her, she gave good care.

I know you're probably thinking, I'm not Mrs. Uddin. I'm not Mary. I'm a nice person. People like me! While I'm sure that's true, doctors don't need to have abject hatred for you in order for your care to suffer. They just need to make personal judgments about you. Let's say, for example, that you're experiencing chest pain. If your doctor perceives you as a complainer or a hysteric, he might not order the EKG that would determine whether you've had a heart attack. He might just chalk the whole experience up to your being whiny. Or take Barbara, the woman we met in the last chapter, whose six-foot-one daughter, Stephanie, weighed 113 pounds. At one point, Barbara got a look at Stephanie's medical records and found that the doctor had made a notation he suspected Stephanie was anorexic. Why, in the face of symptoms such as bloody diarrhea, would he think her weight loss was caused by anorexia? Years later, Barbara and her daughter Stephanie realized that it was basically because the doctor thought they were being hysterical. There was something about them, or something about the doctor, or a combination of the two, that made the doctor not believe her. Thankfully, they did eventually find a doctor who took them seriously, did the proper tests, diagnosed Stephanie with ulcerative colitis, and got her the right treatment. But Stephanie suffered for a decade because her doctor didn't trust her.

There are other reasons that your doctor might not like you. I know doctors hate to hear this, but there's a whole body of evidence showing that physicians make snap judgments about patients based on their gender, the color of their skin, or the size of their body. Let's start with gender. Every February, on Go Red for Women Day, we're reminded that when a man walks into the emergency room with chest pain, doctors are much more likely to take him seriously and check him out for a heart attack than when a woman walks in with the same complaint. In her book *Medical Myths That Can Kill You,* Dr. Nancy Snyderman describes how when she was a medical student doing a rotation in the emergency room, a middle-aged woman walked in with chest pain. The senior doctor asked Dr. Snyderman and her fellow students what it could be. They all eagerly offered up various diagnoses, and he disagreed with all of them. His explanation? "She could be hysterical," he quietly told them. He then gave the woman some antacids and sent her home.

She walked out of the emergency room to her car and dropped dead in the parking lot.

The title of the chapter in which Dr. Snyderman tells this story is "Myth #3: Doctors Don't Play Favorites," and it's aptly named. The truth is, doctors do play favorites—or, to put it another way, doctors take certain patients more seriously than others. As Dr. Snyderman concluded, "To this day, I believe that had a man come into our ER with the same symptoms that this female patient had, the ER doc would have pegged heart disease as the most likely diagnosis." Even after a heart attack, the differences in how men and women are treated continue, with women being less likely to receive beta-blockers, ACE inhibitors, and aspirin, all treatments known to improve survival after a heart attack. This helps explain why women are twice as likely as men to die within the first few weeks after suffering a heart attack.

In an effort to document bias against women in the medical system, researchers in Canada set up a sneaky experiment in which they arranged for two patients with arthritis in the knee, one male and one female, to visit seventy-one doctors. Both patients were comparable in every respect except gender: they were sixty-seven years old, X-rays and physical exams showed that they had the same degree of arthritis, and neither was obese. When the man and woman visited the doctors, they gave the same medical history: they'd been in pain for six months, they experienced pain especially when going up stairs, they couldn't walk for more than twenty to thirty minutes before they had to sit down, and a cortisone shot and physiotherapy hadn't helped. The study coordinators instructed the patients to bring up the option of knee-replacement surgery if the doctor didn't mention it.

Since the only difference between these patients was their gender, you would expect the doctors to offer them the same options for treatment, including knee-replacement surgery, an expensive and very effective option for osteoarthritis of the knee when nothing else works. But the orthopedic surgeons in the study were twenty-two times more likely to recommend knee-replacement surgery for the male patient than for the female patient. The family doctors weren't quite so bad; they were only twice as likely to recommend knee replacements for men than for women. There was no medical reason to recommend knee-replacement surgery more often for men, as the surgery can be a good option for either gender. The authors concluded, "Gender bias may contribute to sex-based disparity in the rates of use of total knee arthroplasty."

This is a fancy way of saying that women sometimes get the shaft at the doctor's office. Other studies have found that women are less likely to get gold-standard treatments for other diseases as well. They're less likely to receive kidney transplants, kidney dialysis, cholesterol-lowering drugs after a heart attack, and cardiac catheterization, a procedure done to examine blood flow and test how well the heart is pumping. Women are also less likely to receive implantable cardiac defibrillators, a device that keeps the heartbeat regular, and less likely to receive lifesaving interventions such as mechanical ventilation in the intensive-care unit.

In all these situations, the doctor is the "gatekeeper," deciding who benefits from these valuable medical interventions and who doesn't, and in each case it was more likely to be men than women. The authors of the knee study explained why this is true: "[Studies have shown] some physicians take women's symptoms less seriously and attribute their symptoms to emotional rather than physical causes and to refer women less often than men for specialty care." Again, I go back to the title of one of the chapters in Dr. Snyderman's book: "Myth #3: Doctors Don't Play Favorites."

Many studies have also shown racial favoritism. In one study, black patients at Veterans Affairs hospitals were less likely than white patients to receive lifesaving treatments such as cardiac catheterization, coronary angioplasty, and coronary bypass surgery. This study is particularly telling, since it wasn't money that made the difference—all the patients, black and white, had the same medical insurance. A similar study, which looked at more than 700,000 patients—all on Medicare—found that African-American patients were less likely to receive cardiac revascularization procedures, which restore the flow of oxygen to the heart. Some studies have found that black and Hispanic women with breast cancer are less likely to receive necessary radiation or chemotherapy treatments. Another study found that black women with breast cancer were nearly four times more likely than white women to have a symptom that wasn't being addressed by the doctor, such as nausea and vomiting, hot flashes, or difficulty sleeping.

In yet another study, researchers looked at the pain pills doctors prescribed to patients who came to the emergency room complaining of back pain or migraines. It turns out that the white patients were more likely than the black patients to walk out with prescriptions for heavy-duty drugs such as OxyContin, Percocet, or Vicodin. The authors of the study explained that there was no medical reason for this discrepancy; all the patients had either back pain or migraines. Their conclusion: physicians worry that patients want opioid drugs like OxyContin to satisfy an addiction, or to sell them. "Prescribing an opioid requires more trust of the patient by the physician," they wrote. "If physicians have greater social distance from minorities, then these physicians may view their patients' reports of pain with less credibility."

In another study, researchers wrote a vignette about a fifty-year-old man who arrived at the emergency room with chest pain. An EKG showed that he'd had a heart attack. The researchers had doctors read this vignette, sometimes pairing it with the photograph of a black man and at other times pairing it with the photograph of a white man. They asked the doctors whether they would give the patient potentially lifesaving drugs that dissolve the clots blocking the flow of blood to the heart. Among the doctors who thought this man was having heart problems, 58 percent were "very likely" to offer clot-busting drugs to the white patients, compared with only 42 percent for the black patients.

As for body size, in one survey taken at a large New York City health-care network, more than 40 percent of the doctors said they had a "negative reaction" to obese patients. In another study, researchers at Rice University wanted to see if doctors spent less time with overweight patients. In a stealthy experiment, they sent fictitious medical charts to 122 doctors. The charts were all for patients with migraine headaches, but some of the patients had normal weight, some were overweight, and others were obese. When the doctors were asked how much time they would spend with each patient, they indicated that they would spend less time with the overweight patients, and even less time with the obese patients: twenty-two minutes with the obese patients, twenty-five minutes with those who were overweight, and thirty-one minutes with patients of average weight. Mind you, there was absolutely no reason for the doctors to spend less time with the fatter patients, since all the patients suffered from the same ailment. In addition to wanting to spend less time with fat patients, the doctors said the slimmer patients were more likely to make them like their job. The doctors also said they'd have more patience with the slimmer patients and less patience with the ones who were fat, and that they had a greater personal desire to help the patients with normal weight than those who were overweight or obese. Finally, to top it all off, the doctors said the overweight and obese patients were more likely to annoy them.

In another study, medical students were more likely to link adjectives such as "worthless," "unpleasant," "bad," "ugly," "awkward," and "unsuccessful" to obese patients than to patients whose weight was normal. Another study found that out of dozens of different categories, physicians ranked obesity number four on the negativity scale, behind drug addiction, alcoholism, and mental illness. Studies have found that 48 percent of nurses felt uncomfortable caring for obese patients; 24 percent said they were "repulsed" by obese people, and 35 percent said they would prefer not to care for obese patients.

So what do all these studies tell you about choosing Dr. Right? *Your* Dr. Right will take *you* seriously. Your Dr. Right won't have preconceived notions about you because you're a woman, or black, or overweight. So how do you know if a doctor has preconceived notions about you? Of course, it won't really work to ask a question like "Hey, Doc, do you have a thing about fat people?" because you won't get an honest answer. Instead, you'll have to rely on your instincts. Dr. Cornelius Flowers, a cardiologist at Emory Hospital, put it simply. "If you feel like you have a doctor who isn't genuinely concerned about you, just get another doctor next time," he told me. Patients should act on their gut instincts, he said. If your gut says a doctor looks down on you or isn't taking you seriously, you're probably right.

SOLUTIONS: HOW TO FIND DR. RIGHT

Dr. Right is someone who trusts your instincts about your own body, believes what you say, communicates well with you, and, as we've seen, actually likes you.

So how do you find this Dr. Right? First of all, look for him or her when you're healthy. When you're sick, you're desperate, and you know what happens when you're desperate to find a mate, right? You often end up settling for the wrong person. The same thing happens with doctors: if you search for Dr. Right when you're ill, you'll take the first white coat you see. In keeping with this romance metaphor, your first step toward finding Dr. Right is to ask your friends to fix you up with doctors they like. Make sure you ask friends whose temperament is similar to yours. If you're an independent kind of person, don't ask a a friend who's more on the passive side for a recommendation. You could end up with a controlling doctor who wants to call all the shots, which may work fine for your friend but not for you.

Once you have a list of possible doctors, start "dating" them until you meet Dr. Right. You can make an appointment for a screening interview. If the doctor won't do this (and many won't), make an appointment for something small. "Just as you would 'do' coffee on a first date instead of a weekend together, so, too, go to the first appointment with a problem of a limited scope, like a mole or a thyroid check," suggests Dr. Vicki Rackner, a surgeon and a patient advocate. You could also ask about a particular medical problem that's been bugging you. Christine Miserandino, a woman with lupus who runs the popular website butyoudontlooksick .com, once had a doctor who wanted her to take painkillers that made her drowsy, even though she had explained to him that she needed to be alert in order to care for her baby. When she interviewed new doctors, she asked them what they would recommend in her situation.

Remember, you're not just marrying the doctor, you're marrying the whole staff, so from the minute you call to make your appointment, take some mental notes. Does it take an inordinate amount of time to get a human being on the line? Is the staff helpful? These are the people you'll be relying on when you wake up one morning sick as a dog, so pay attention. In the waiting room, do you see a lot of pharmaceutical reps? They're easy to spot: they'll be the good-looking young people in suits dragging suitcases behind them. These attractive, perky people try to get your doctor to prescribe their company's drugs by giving them goodies like free lunches. This might mean that your doctor's choice of drugs will be based on what the pharma reps tell her, rather than on her own sound medical judgment. Watch the reps while you're in the waiting room—if your doctor's running late and the rep gets in before the patients, that's particularly disturbing.

Once inside the examining room for this "first date" with your prospective Dr. Right, be aware of her demeanor. The doctor's focus should be completely on you, even if she's busy (and what doctor isn't?). While in the examining room, you should feel like your problem is the most important issue at that moment. Dr. John Santa, director of the Consumer Reports Health Ratings Center, says to pay close attention to a doctor's body language. "Does the physician look at you directly, sit down, and slow down?" he asks. Even if she comes highly recommended and has all the credentials in the world, if you feel she's not focused on you, get another doctor. A lack of focus for a minor ailment might not be a big deal, but a lack of focus for a serious medical problem could kill you. Also, pay close attention to how well you and the doctor communicate. Do you feel comfortable with her? Do you feel like she's dominating the conversation, or do the two of you seem to have a good back-and-forth?

There's an exception to this good-rapport rule. The rule can—and sometimes should—be broken for a specialist with whom you'll have a short-term relationship. Once I went to see a podiatrist who had all the communication skills of a potted plant. Since I saw him just twice, I didn't care so much. He came highly recommended for his surgical skills, and I just needed to get some chunks of wood yanked out of my foot. (Note to self: wear shoes when walking in the backyard.) In this situation, what's important is how often a physician performs a certain procedure—once a week? once a month? less frequently? Compare the answers from different physicians. You want someone who does this surgery on a regular basis, not someone for whom this is a side job. This rule also applies if you've been diagnosed with an unusual disease, such as a rare cancer. You want someone who's seen many, many patients like you, not someone who dallies in your disease. To get a true specialist for an unusual problem, you may have to compromise somewhat on communication skills in order to get a physician who has the necessary experience.

However, for your primary-care physician—a pediatrician or family doctor or internist—you really do need an excellent communicator. At your "first date" appointment, ask the doctor a couple of specific questions. Find out, for example, if she's always available during office hours, or if it may be necessary for you to see another doctor in the practice, or perhaps a nurse practitioner or a physician's assistant. Also find out how she handles simple questions that don't require an appointment. Can you email her? How quickly are phone calls returned? What happens if you get sick on an evening, weekend, or holiday? And find out how in tune you are with this doctor, medically speaking. If you're really into alternative medicine, you want a doctor who believes in it, too. I once interviewed a very religious woman who said that she wanted her doctor to pray with her when she was sick. If something like that is important to you, ask about it.

If you like a doctor, invest a few minutes in checking her out on the Internet to avoid any future surprises. First, Google your prospective dream doctor to make sure she's not on the FBI's most-wanted list, or the author of a "How to Make Weapons of Mass Destruction" blog. Then, once you've made sure there's nothing big and scary out there, do one more check to make sure the doctor hasn't been disciplined by the state medical licensing board for amputating the wrong leg or having sex with patients. (See page 179 for a list of these websites.) There are also doctor-rating sites on the Internet, but I'd use them with caution. They're often pretty meaningless because there are only a few comments for any one doctor; a couple of angry (or delighted) reviews don't mean much, as the former could have been written by a disgruntled former employee and the latter by the doctor's mother. However, I'd pay attention if many people voice the same specific criticism. For example, fifteen people saying "Dr. Smith showed up drunk to my appointment!" is a big red flag.

In the end, as with a spouse, you want a doctor you trust and feel good about. It's perfectly okay during your selection process to reject doctors simply because there's something about them you don't like. As Dr. Rackner puts it, "There are lots of nice people out there, but you would not want to marry most of them."

So let's say you've found your Dr. Right and you're in medical bliss for many years, but something happens that makes you unhappy with your doctor. Many of us have a really hard time doing this, but it's perfectly okay to fire Dr. Wrong. I don't mean you should willy-nilly go doctor hopping when something isn't perfect, but if a physician isn't taking care of your medical needs you can and should look elsewhere. I know this is tough—it's hard to leave a hairdresser you've been going to for a long time, let alone a doctor—but sometimes you just have to do it.

My little sister is a great example of someone who had a hard time firing her doctor. Julia and her husband, John, have struggled with infertility for years. After several miscarriages and multiple rounds of in vitro fertilization, we were over the moon when she finally became pregnant five years ago and gave birth to my darling niece and nephew, Charlotte and Aidan. When Julia and John decided that they wanted to expand their family, they went back to the same fertility doctor who'd helped them get the twins. After two rounds of failed in vitro, Dr. IVF told Julia she'd hit the end of the road. She said that at age forty-one, my sister was clearly too old to get pregnant. But Julia had done her homework. On the Internet she'd read about a new fertility treatment that her doctor hadn't mentioned, so she asked if it might work for her. Absolutely not, Dr. IVF told her. When Julia pressed for a reason she couldn't try this new procedure, the doctor told her it was because she has high blood pressure and this new procedure would require her to take birth-control pills, which can increase blood pressure.

Deflated, Julia left the doctor's office. But my sister's a crackerjack lawyer who's accustomed to winning in the courtroom, and she wasn't about to be defeated that easily. She looked up this procedure online again to see if her doctor was right. Her doctor was wrong. Julia found several studies by fertility specialists who had done this new procedure successfully *without* using birth-control pills. She also found doctors who thought the procedure could safely be performed on women with high blood pressure who took birth-control pills as long as they were monitored carefully. Sure that she'd found the answer to her problem, Julia excitedly went back to Dr. IVF with her newfound information. But Dr. IVF persisted in claiming that this procedure would never work for Julia. "Do I have any other options?" my sister asked desperately. No, there were none, the doctor told her. She'd have to give up.

Devastated, Julia and her husband left the examining room. On their way out, they heard a voice. "Psst," it said. "Come in here." Looking around to see where the voice was coming from, Julia and John saw a nurse in an examining room hiding behind the door. "Quick, come in," the nurse whispered, closing the door behind them. "I could lose my job if the doctor knew I was talking to you. But I have to tell you that there are well-respected doctors who will do this procedure on you. Dr. IVF won't do it because, well, we just don't do that treatment here. The head of our practice doesn't believe it works, and so none of the doctors do it. But there's a fertility specialist down the street who does it all the time. Go see her." John and Julia wrote down the other doctor's name and, after promising never to mention the conversation, slipped out of the room.

"It was like something out of a spy novel," Julia told me the next day. "It was crazy. What do you think I should do?"

"What do you mean, what do I think you should do?" I asked her. "You should go see that other doctor."

"But I don't want to leave Dr. IVF. She's been so good to us. If it weren't for her, we wouldn't have Charlotte and Aidan," she said.

What was this—my killer lawyer sister getting all mushy on me?

I explained to Julia that while I understood her sentimental attachment to the doctor who had given her the twins, Dr. IVF, who had been Dr. Right for a long time, was now clearly Dr. Wrong. "She told you she won't do the procedure, and there's nothing else left for you to try. Why not go see the other doctor? You don't have to try the new procedure, but you could at least listen to what she has to say. What have you got to lose?" I asked. "Plus, it's a little disturbing that Dr. IVF told you there were absolutely no options left when there are legitimate doctors who would disagree with her."

Julia did go to see the other doctor, who said that she was a great candidate for the new procedure, and she's trying it now. After the visit with this doctor, Julia couldn't believe what her former doctor had done. "I get it that Dr. IVF didn't want to do this procedure—that's her prerogative," my sister said. "But why didn't she tell me that there were other doctors who would do it? Why didn't she refer me to them?"

My sister's experience illustrates one of the minimums you should expect from Dr. Right: she should lay out all the legitimate treatments to you even if she doesn't offer them herself. Even if this doctor didn't want to perform this particular procedure—and she might have had good reasons for not wanting to do it—she should at least have informed Julia that other well-respected doctors did do it. Julia shouldn't have had to learn about these other doctors from a nurse whispering behind closed doors.

As my sister's experience shows, you should fire a doctor who jeopardizes your care by not telling you all the options. Another reason to consider firing a doctor immediately is his or her failure to give you the care you need when you're severely ill. Dr. Joan Harrold, an internist and a co-author of *Handbook for Mortals: Guidance for People Facing Serious Illness,* advises that if you're sick and call your doctor you should get a phone call back from the doctor or the nurse within ninety minutes, and you should expect to be seen in person that day if you're seriously ill and need a new prescription or test. Another reason for instant dismissal is disrespectful treatment by a doctor. Dr. Jerome Groopman says a reader wrote to tell him that when she asked an orthopedic surgeon a question about her care, his response was "Since when did you get an MD?" That kind of response, Dr. Groopman told me, "is just about a deal-breaker." Another possible deal-breaker: when your doctor dismisses your observations about your own health. Debra Roter, a behavioral scientist at Johns Hopkins and a co-author of *Doctors Talking with Patients,* has a friend whose doctor wanted her to take a certain drug. "She told him she'd taken the drug before and it hadn't worked for her," Roter says. "But her doctor wanted her to try it anyway. He didn't give her any credibility." Her friend realized that she was with Dr. Wrong, and she fired him.

Sometimes your doctor will do something that's not a deal-breaker but is bad enough that you'll want to put her on notice in your own mind. For example, if your doctor doesn't explain things in terms you can understand, and she does this on more than one occasion, and keeps doing it even when you say you don't get it, that's a red flag that you should think about taking your business elsewhere. "Patients should have a basic expectation that they're going to be provided information they need in terms they understand," says Diane Pinakiewicz, the president of the National Patient Safety Foundation. This means getting information that you can understand when you're sick and your brain's not functioning at its best.

Also, if your doctor's office takes too long to call you with test results, take note. If this happens repeatedly, it might not be a random occurrence but a sign that the office is seriously disorganized. How long is too long? Several doctors I talked to said that you should get test results within forty-eight hours of having the test, or sooner if it's urgent. When you go for the test, ask when the results will be back. Simple lab work is often done in a day. More complicated tests can take a week or longer.

If your doctor doesn't explain the side effects of the drugs she prescribed, that's another red flag that perhaps she's not the doctor for you. You shouldn't expect her to recite every single possible problem with every drug—that might take all day—but she should tell you the especially dangerous ones ("You might get a stroke from this medication") and very common side effects ("This drug might make your mouth dry").

Here are a few more reasons to consider firing your doctor. If you repeatedly have to spend inordinate amounts of time in the waiting room (more than fifteen minutes or so), that's a problem, especially if there are no apologies or assurances that it won't happen again.

When you get into the examining room and you feel like the doctor is rushing you, you might not want to fire her on the spot—she may just be having a bad day. But keep your guard up: if this happens again and again, you might need to be in a rush to get a new doctor. Finally, if a staff member—and not the doctor—calls with abnormal test results, mentally put this doctor on "maybe" status. Physicians I've talked to agree: when the news is bad, you should get a call from the doctor, not a nurse or a secretary. Ditto if the results are normal but there are still decisions to be made about how you'll be treated.

A good rule of thumb here is you should demand the same good service from a doctor that you expect from people in other areas of your life. Dr. Harrold told me that she got stuck in the snow once and had to call AAA. "A lovely gentleman got on the phone and said to me, 'What can I do? I'm here for you,' " she recalled. "If I can get that from AAA, I should get that from my physician's office."

When Your Doctor Fires *You*

Amy didn't have to fire her doctor; her doctor fired her first.

Amy came home one day after picking her children up from school to find a certified letter in the mailbox. It was from her internist, who told her that he would no longer be able to see her and she had thirty days to find a new physician. Amy called the doctor's office. Was he moving out of town? Retiring? Nope. He just didn't want to see her anymore. Amy felt hurt, and she wasn't sure she could find a doctor she'd like in just one month. As a cancer survivor, she needed to have a doctor right at hand. "I was more than ticked off," she told me. "I'd been with him for almost ten years. It was a lot of stress finding a new doctor I could trust."

What made her doctor so angry that he ditched her? I asked Amy. She pondered the question for a moment. "Well, I like to ask a lot of questions, and he did seem kind of impatient with me," she recalled. "And when I brought in printouts from the Internet he didn't seem to like that." And how did she feel when her doctor became impatient with her questions, or looked at her stack of papers with disdain? Not very good, she told me. In fact, now that she thought about it, she hadn't really been very happy with him for quite some time. Even though it would be a pain to find another doctor—and jarring to get that letter in the mail— Amy realized that her doctor had done her a favor by firing her. She realized that she should have fired him long ago.

CONCLUSION: HE'S JUST NOT THAT INTO YOU

Dr. Howard Beckman, a professor of medicine at the University of Rochester, studies the doctor-patient relationship and is one very self-aware guy. He knows precisely what kind of patients he just can't stand, for instance, and he gives them to someone else. "For example, I really don't like passive-aggressive people," he explains. "A lot of other doctors don't like taking care of drug addicts. But drug addicts don't bother me, so sometimes I'll offer a trade. I'll take their drug addict, and they'll take my passive-aggressive."

Occasionally Dr. Beckman has a patient he just doesn't like and he can't figure out why. He remembers one in particular from early in his career. "It was really quite dramatic," he recalls. "This gentleman was a new patient, and I started taking a medical history from him, and I became very agitated. I just didn't want to listen to him. I just felt distaste for him. I really didn't like him." Halfway through the patient's description of his problems, Dr. Beckman interrupted him. "I said to him, 'I'm sorry, this just is not going to work out for us, and I don't want to waste your time if I'm not going to do the best job. Is it okay if I find you someone else in the practice?' I found him another doctor, and they did just fine together."

What exactly bothered you about this patient? I asked him. Dr. Beckman paused. "I wish I could tell you, but I don't know. I've told this story many times, and I still don't know. All I know is that I didn't like him, and it was a very clear response."

"Aha!" I said. "It's just like Miranda in *Sex and the City*!"

Dr. Beckman paused again. "Excuse me?" he said.

Dr. Beckman, it turns out, isn't a big *Sex and the City* fan. But I am, and I know the "he's just not that into you" episode by heart. One evening Miranda's out with her friends Samantha, Charlotte, Carrie, and Carrie's boyfriend, Berger. Miranda tells them how she was out with this great guy the other night and she invited him up to her apartment after dinner (wink, wink), and he declined. Carrie and the other girlfriends console Miranda, offering all sorts of explanations for why this man didn't go up to her apartment. Berger shocks the group of gals by predicting that Miranda will never hear from this man again. "He's just not that into you," Berger tells her. Miranda is taken aback for a minute, then reconsiders. "Wow, he's just not that into me. He's just not that into me," she says. "I love it. That's the most liberating thing I've ever heard."

If you take away the part about the possibility of sex in the apartment, there's a kernel of truth here about relationships between doctors and patients. Feeling that your doctor gets you—that the two of you connect—is really important. It will help get you better care. As Dr. Levinson explains, "If a doctor connects with a patient, they might take longer with the patient. They might be a little more patient with the patient. We do it because we're human beings. It's not necessarily conscious." The lack of a connection, of a "chattiness" with your doctor, is a bad sign, and reason enough to look elsewhere, because a doctor who doesn't like you won't explain your diagnosis and treatment plan carefully, won't answer your questions thoroughly, and won't go to bat for you when your insurance gives you a hard time.

It's up to you to know when your doctor's not that into you, when she doesn't mesh with you for whatever reason. Certain relationships, whether romantic or medical, just aren't meant to be. Dr. Beckman didn't have a reason when he "divorced" his patient and found a new doctor for him, but he did it because he knew he wouldn't communicate well with someone he didn't like very much. As I said, Dr. Beckman is one very self-aware guy, and you can't rely on other doctors to do the same. It's up to you to leave and go find Dr. Right.

Once I heard Dr. Beckman's story, I wondered if I could be wrong about my mother's internist. Maybe he wasn't sexist—or maybe that was only part of why he'd missed my mother's diagnosis so egregiously. I started to picture my mom in his office. I'm sure she bubbled over with enthusiasm about her work. In addition to seeing clients in her social work practice, she's a professor at a prestigious graduate school and also travels extensively to help care for her eleven grandchildren, who are spread across the country. I can just picture this guy thinking, What's *with* this woman? I'm exhausted just listening to her! (Or, as my mom puts it, "It was easy to write off this crazy lady.") Her doctor's first impulse was to conclude that if this grandma would just take it easy her blood pressure would go down, and this conclusion probably clouded all other explanations for her high blood pressure. But this doctor just didn't *get* my mother. He didn't get that her constant activity isn't what makes her suffer. In fact, it's what keeps her alive.

The day after her "he's just not that into you" epiphany, Miranda spreads the gospel to two lovelorn women. "Excuse me, but I couldn't help but hear your conversation," Miranda tells them. "He's just not that into you. So move on."

Now, if we could just get Miranda to tell that to Elaine.

Final Checklist: Five Steps for Finding Dr. Right

1. **Take the doctor on a test drive.** Interview prospective doctors to see if you like the doctor and the staff. Some doctors won't do a "meet and greet," so instead go in with a small problem and see how she handles it.

2. **Keep your eyes open during your visit.** Is the office full of frustrated patients who have been waiting for hours? Is the staff attentive? Does the doctor rush you through the visit? Does she interrupt you halfway through your sentences? Are there pharmaceutical reps getting in to see her before you?

3. **Ask how your doctor handles illnesses that occur after hours.** We don't get sick on schedule. What's the plan if you need your doctor on a Saturday, or at midnight? Is she or one of her partners on call, or will she refer you to an emergency room? While you're checking this out, ask whether during normal office hours you'll see your doctor or one of her partners. The pediatric practice that I initially chose for my daughters had nine doctors and three different locations. I often ended up seeing a doctor I'd never met before. We switched to a practice that had only two pediatricians.

4. **Google your doctor.** If your doctor has posted pictures of her-

self drunk and naked, that might be nice to know. If she's been convicted of a felony or sued repeatedly for lopping off the wrong body part, that would be good to know, too.

5. **Do a gut check: Do you like this doctor? Do you think she likes you?** Whether it's a doctor, a date, or a co-worker, we all have pretty good inner barometers for whether we like them or they like us. Listen to that voice. Don't see someone if you don't feel comfortable with her, or if you suspect she isn't comfortable with you. You could be depending on this person through some pretty tough times, and you want to enjoy a good relationship.

CHAPTER THREE

Don't Leave a Doctor's Appointment Saying "Huh?"

Often—I would say at least once a week—someone asks me for advice about a medical problem. The other day at CNN, I was about three minutes away from going on air and running to the studio when a co-worker accosted me in the hallway. "Hey, Elizabeth," he said. "My daughter's really short, and we're considering putting her on human growth hormone. What do you think?"

What do I think? Yikes! That's what I think! Whether or not to put your child on hormones is not a discussion to be had in the hallway, in three minutes, with someone who isn't even a doctor. Another colleague once wanted to know if I thought her mother should go on hormone replacement therapy. Someone else asked me about chemotherapy for his father's cancer. I've always wondered, Why are all these people coming to me? Why aren't they asking their doctor these questions? Or, if they are asking their doctor, why are they leaving their appointments sufficiently dissatisfied with the answer so that they then feel the need to seek counsel from me? What's wrong with this picture?

DR. PAUL KONOWITZ AND HIS AMAZINGLY DISAPPOINTING DOCTOR'S APPOINTMENT

Most of us love to get compliments when we lose weight, but a few years back when friends and co-workers told Dr. Paul Konowitz how slim he looked, he'd smile and say thanks, but inside his heart was sinking.

It had all started out with an irritating taste in his mouth. Dr. Konowitz didn't think much of it, but the next thing he knew, painful blisters started appearing in his mouth. "Imagine that feeling when you burn your mouth on hot pizza—now magnify it by about one hundred," he says. At first it was somewhat painful to eat, and then it became extremely painful, so he started eating as little as possible. Dr. Konowitz, an ear, nose, and throat doctor at the Massachusetts Eye and Ear Infirmary and a clinical instructor at Harvard Medical School, had seen viruses wreak this kind of havoc in his patients' mouths, so he took some antiviral medications. When those didn't work, he asked a friend to biopsy a few of his blisters. The results were worse than he feared. Dr. Konowitz had pemphigus vulgaris, an autoimmune disease in which the body attacks itself, creating blisters on any surface, like the mouth, that's lined with mucous membranes. He remembered learning about this disease during his medical training. "During my dermatology rotation as a medical student, my professor proclaimed that there were two dermatologic problems that you especially never wanted to develop. I can't remember the name of the first one. The second one was pemphigus vulgaris," Dr. Konowitz wrote in an essay about his experience. "The lining of my nose, throat, and mouth were basically just sloughing off."

Dr. Konowitz immediately set out to get treatment. His doctor prescribed high doses of steroids, which helped to get rid of the blisters, but the steroids also ravaged his muscles and made it nearly impossible for him to sleep. He became so irritable and weak that he couldn't work, so his doctor gave him drugs that allowed him to decrease the steroid doses. But these new drugs suppressed the immune system, leaving him vulnerable to every little bug that was in the air. He caught a herpes infection in his esophagus, the tube that takes food from the throat to the stomach. In unrelenting pain from the herpes sores up and down his esophagus, he ended up in the hospital. The gastroenterologist on call performed tests, discharged him, and told him to follow up with an office visit.

Dr. Konowitz had high hopes for this follow-up appointment. He was still in pain from the herpes sores and was really hoping the gastroenterologist would know what to do. His wife, who is also a physician, took the day off so that she could go with him. But something strange happened at this doctor's appointment. "We talked to the doctor for about fifteen minutes, and then he just kind of got up and left the room. The appointment was over," Dr. Konowitz recalls. The doctor had given the Konowitzes no treatment plan, no directions, no suggestions, no nothing. "My wife and I looked at each other and said, 'What was that all about?' We didn't know anything more than when we went in."

Dr. Konowitz left that doctor's office, and later had to call him up "yelling and screaming." He ordered his doctor to confer with his colleagues and ask what they recommended, which the doctor did. Eventually, the herpes sores went away on their own without treatment, but Dr. Konowitz will never forget that useless doctor's appointment. And if a useless doctor's appointment can happen to two physicians, it can happen to you.

WHAT THE STUDIES SAY

Earlier, I asked what was wrong with this picture, why so many people were leaving the doctor's office so full of unanswered questions that they were turning to me—someone who's not a doctor—for medical advice. Here's the answer: eighteen and twenty-three.

Allow me to explain.

Eighteen minutes is how long the average doctor's appointment lasts. Did you ever have an eighteen-minute business meeting that yielded useful results? Probably not. So how can you be expected to have a thoughtful discussion about the most important issue in your life—your health—in just eighteen minutes? Unless it's something extremely simple, eighteen minutes just isn't enough time to tell your doctor what's wrong, have him ask you questions, do a physical exam, think through your problem, come up with a diagnosis and a treatment plan, present these to you in a coherent way, and then allow you to ask questions. (This eighteen minutes comes from a 2001 study; my guess is visits now are even shorter.)

Now, about twenty-three: that's the number of seconds patients talk, on average, before the doctor interrupts. That's right—you'll be explaining your problem, and wham, twenty-three seconds into your story the doctor will cut in with a question or a comment. Dr. Howard Beckman, the professor at the University of Rochester I mentioned in chapter 2, actually documented these interruptions when he taped doctors with their patients. He calls it "redirecting," because the doctor is making you lose your train of thought, directing your attention away from what you, the patient, think is most important. So, for example, you might be talking about the headaches you've been having, and after twenty-three seconds your doctor interrupts and asks you to describe these headaches: is the pain sharp or dull, and is it on one side or all over? You answer the doctor's questions, he whips out his pad and hands you a prescription for your headache, and suddenly he's walking out the door. But because the doctor interrupted your story, you didn't get a chance to mention that you've been having chest pain, too. That chest pain is actually more important than your headaches, but you never had a chance to mention it. Or maybe you're forced to mention the chest pain as the doctor's about to leave the room. "The doctor blames the patients, and says, oh, those stupid people, they always bring the important stuff up at the end," Beckman told me. But that's what happens when the doctor interrupts.

On top of all this, $18 + 23 = 5$. Allow me to explain once again. For a research project, Sherrie Kaplan, an associate dean of the School of Medicine at the University of California, Irvine, tape-recorded patients at their doctor's appointments and counted the number of questions the patients asked. On average, the patients asked only five questions per appointment—and that included "Where's the ladies' room?" and "Do you validate parking?" How in the world can you truly understand something as complex as your health when you're asking fewer than five real questions? But it's not surprising, considering that your appointment is only eighteen minutes long and the doctor interrupts you after twenty-three seconds. "Doctors are increasingly on a time-pressured schedule, needing to be efficient because that's how our system rewards people these days, so when the doctor asks at the end of a visit if you have any questions, he's looking at his watch and the waiting room is full of people, so you know the answer is 'No,' " Kaplan says. Plus, you're probably not feeling well to begin with *and* you're sitting there in a paper gown, so you're not exactly at your intellectual best. "I tell people, imagine taking a math test in a johnny," Kaplan says, using an old-fashioned term for examining-room garb.

As you can see, in so many different ways you're set up for failure when you go to the doctor. "Most of us go to an appointment unprepared," Kaplan says. "We show up and say, 'Doctor, take good care of me.' " Kaplan says we all need to stop being passive and start practicing what she calls "planned patienthood." Planned patienthood means thinking through what you want to get out of the appointment before you even set foot in the doctor's office. Planned patienthood means walking into the examining room with a list of questions. Planned patienthood means remembering what issues are important even when the doctor interrupts you. It means asking every last question you have and walking out with a clear idea of what you need to do right now in order to get better. In short, planned patienthood means getting the most out of those eighteen minutes you have with the doctor.

When Kaplan noticed that patients asked so few questions at the doctor's office, she knew she had to do something. What do you do when your tennis game isn't going well? You get a coach. So Kaplan decided to start coaching patients. With the doctors' consent, she actually went to waiting rooms, found people reading outdated copies of *Ladies' Home Journal,* and dragged them into a conference room for coaching.

Kaplan told the patients to do some planning for their upcoming appointment. What did they hope to get out of it? Did they have a plan for success? For example, if the patient was a diabetic, the coach would ask her to think about glucose levels. Had they been staying under control, or had they been spiking? If the levels were too high, was it because the patient was having a tough time sticking to the doctor's plan? If so, what could be changed about the plan? How would she get back in touch with the doctor if the changes weren't working? Should she just call and leave a message or should she make a new appointment, or perhaps send an email?

Kaplan's coaching paid off. A study of diabetics who were coached showed that their blood-sugar levels were under better control than those of diabetics who didn't receive coaching.

SOLUTION: GET IT DUN!

"What I really want is for my patients to be prepared like a Boy Scout," says Dr. Dana Frank, an internist at Johns Hopkins. A Boy Scout doesn't waste precious time, particularly when he has only eighteen minutes. A Boy Scout would never have a conversation like this:

DOCTOR: Tell me, what medications are you taking?
PATIENT: Hmm, something pink and something yellow once a day. Or twice a day. Or something like that.
DOCTOR: And how about your family history—anyone have heart disease?

PATIENT: Mom did. Or maybe she had diabetes. Or toe fungus. One of those.

DOCTOR: Okay, let's move on. You had blood tests with Dr. Jones last month. My office never got the results. What were the tests for?

PATIENT: Hmm, something that begins with a C. Cholesterol. Cold sores. Cancer . . . Something like that.

To be prepared like a Boy Scout, bring to your appointment a list of everything you're taking—prescription medicines, over-the-counter drugs, herbs, and supplements. "It's surprising and unfortunate how much time is wasted when that list isn't together," says Dr. Adam Dimitrov, an internist in Baltimore. You can also just put everything you're taking in a bag and hand the bag to your doctor. And, speaking of being prepared, always make sure you have your insurance card with you. (It should always be in your wallet in case of emergencies.) To make for a more efficient appointment, bring some notes with you. First, bring in a list of the top three concerns you'd like to have addressed during the appointment to keep you focused on what's important. Also, if your medical history is complicated, jot down a few notes about your medical history, including all relevant treatments, surgeries, and procedures. It will really save time if you can just hand this list to the doctor rather than hemming and hawing your way through it. You should also bring in test results from other doctors' offices. "Don't count on another physician taking the time to send your results to your current doctor; even if they do, it may end up sitting on someone's desk," Dr. Konowitz says. To get results from one doctor so that you can give them to another, just ask to have them faxed, emailed, or snail-mailed to you directly. You can also ask a doctor to give you a note for another doctor explaining what treatments and tests you've had and other facts about your medical history.

The "Get It DUN!" Plan

Let's freeze Dr. Konowitz and his wife in the moment where they were looking at each other dumbfounded because they'd come to the end of that appointment with his gastroenterologist having accomplished nothing. What could they have done differently to get a better result? Dr. Konowitz himself has the answer. "Maybe it would have helped if at the beginning of the appointment I'd said I needed a clear plan for what to do," he told me. "We needed a plan, next steps, and a time frame for what to do if I didn't get better."

A plan . . . next steps . . . and a time frame. In short, Dr. Konowitz needed to get his business done—or DUN! That's an easy way to remember the three things you'd better know when you walk out of a doctor's appointment: you want to know your **d**iagnosis; you want to **u**nderstand the plan to get you better; and you want to know the **n**ext steps you need to put that plan into action.

Let's start with the **diagnosis.** Getting your doctor to give you a specific diagnosis may not be as simple as it sounds. Let's say Mrs. Smith has gained a lot of weight lately and has been feeling sluggish. Her doctor does a blood test and tells her, "Something's wrong with your thyroid, Mrs. Smith." That's not a diagnosis. It's vague and mushy, and she shouldn't settle for it. She needs the actual diagnosis, which in this case is hypothyroidism, and she needs to know how to spell it correctly. "I write down a patient's diagnosis, because I know people will want to Google it," Dr. Konowitz says. If your doctor doesn't write it down for you, write it down yourself and show it to him to make sure you have it right.

Once you know the diagnosis, make sure you **understand your treatment plan.** Staying with our example, let's say Mrs. Smith's doctor prescribes a synthetic thyroid hormone. Mrs. Smith should get more details: How long will she be on this drug? Are there side effects she should watch out for? Is this the only treatment, or should she be doing something else in addition?

Once she understands the plan to get her healthy, Mrs. Smith needs to find out **next steps,** or what she should do after she leaves the doctor's office. How will she know if the treatment isn't working? Should she expect to feel better in a few days? A few weeks? If she doesn't feel better in that time period, what should she do? Should she call back and leave a message with a nurse? And if the pills do work does she need to come back at a certain point to see the doctor for a follow-up visit?

This "next steps" part is really crucial. Without it, you might make a critical error, as I once did. It happened when my oldest daughter had her first ear infection. The pediatrician prescribed an antibiotic for ten days, and off I went without asking any questions. A day passed, then two, three, four. My baby still wasn't getting better. I figured this was normal, and that it would just take a while for the antibiotics to kick in. Finally, after a week, I took her back to the pediatrician. He looked inside her ears, and they were still infected. The pediatrician immediately switched her to another antibiotic and told me to call in two days if it didn't seem to be working. "Two days?" I asked. "The antibiotics should work in two days?" Yes, he explained. If a child's ear infection hasn't improved after two days on an antibiotic, it means the medicine might not be working and you need to try another one. I had no idea. I had thought it would take a lot longer than that for an antibiotic to work. I felt terrible. If I had just asked one question—"How long should it take this medicine to work?"—I could have saved my baby several days of pain.

Of course, the best way to plan all this is to write down everything. During your appointment with the doctor, write down the diagnosis, the treatment plan, and the next steps on a "Get it DUN!" worksheet, which you'll find on page 180 of the appendix, along with a website where you can print out more worksheets. I also have a sample of a "Get It DUN!" conversation between an empowered patient and a doctor, and her completed "Get It DUN!" worksheet so you can see how it's done.

SPECIAL INSTRUCTIONS FOR COMPLICATED PROBLEMS

If you have a complicated medical problem, you'd better be prepared not just like any old Boy Scout but like a *really smart* Boy Scout. With a major medical issue, being disorganized could put your health in jeopardy. Christine Miserandino, the young woman we met in chapter 2 who has lupus and runs a popular website called butyoudon'tlooksick.com, has explained to me how important it is for a patient with a complex disease to be able to manage her own illness. First, ask yourself what symptoms are bringing you to the doctor. Have they become more severe, less severe, or changed in any way since the last time you saw the doctor? Does anything in particular trigger your symptoms? Does anything make them feel better? Then think about your diagnoses and treatments. What other treatments have you tried, and did they work? If your doctor recommended treatments or medications at the last visit, did they work? Are there any new treatments you've heard of and would like to ask your doctor about?

To help you organize your thoughts when you have a complex medical problem, I've put a worksheet on page 184 of the appendix.

WHEN THINGS GO WRONG: LONG WAITS
AND RUSHED DOCTORS

Let's go back to our dating analogy. Even when you've found Mr. or Ms. Right, it's not always smooth sailing. There are bound to be bumps in the road, and the same is true with your health care. Even with the best doctor in the world, something is sure to go wrong. You might need an appointment quickly and the secretary tells you the doctor is booked for the next six months. Or, when you arrive for the appointment, you might spend three hours in the waiting room. Or, when you have a question, you might end up playing phone tag with the doctor or nurse for days on end. It's important to learn how to deal with all of these problems.

First, let's attack the issue of having to wait a long time to get an appointment with a doctor. The other day my friend Renee called to make a doctor's appointment for her elderly mother, who was lying in bed in excruciating pain from a degenerative disk in her back. The appointment secretary told Renee the doctor couldn't see her for another five days. Renee was devastated. I told her to call back and push for an earlier appointment. The secretary she spoke with is the lowest-ranking person in the office. A "wait five days" from her doesn't *really* mean you have to wait five days. I told Renee to ask to speak with a nurse or the office manager to get an appointment sooner. It worked; the doctor saw her mother the next day and prescribed medication. Renee's persistence saved her mother four days of pain.

When you get the nurse or the office manager on the phone, be ready to give a good explanation for why you need to be seen quickly. The goal here, Dr. Konowitz says, is to make them feel sorry for you. "Let them feel your pain; you want them to have sympathy for you and your sense of urgency," he told me. This means a lot of details. While a member of Dr. Konowitz's staff might not clear time in his schedule for someone with a sore throat, "If he said he had a sore throat and it felt like his throat was closing, this might indicate a more serious issue," Dr. Konowitz says. And remember, don't get angry. "Be polite but persistent," advises Dr. John Santa, the director of the Consumer Reports Health Ratings Center.

When being polite doesn't work, Dr. Konowitz has this advice: go a little crazy. One of his patients did just that when she couldn't get in to see him on short notice. She actually called a local TV station to complain. True story! When I wrote about this on cnn.com, doctors, nurses, and office staff went berserk in the comments section under my story, howling about the inappropriateness of such a tactic. Inappropriate as it might have been, it worked. A reporter from the news show called the public-relations folks at the hospital where Dr. Konowitz works, and the PR person called Dr. Konowitz, who made sure he saw the woman that day. If going crazy like this isn't your style, Dr. Konowitz advises that you just go to the doctor's office and plunk yourself in the waiting room. Sooner or later, someone might take pity on you and get you in to see the doctor.

Sometimes you don't need to see a doctor that day, but you do need to get in relatively quickly, like in the next week or two. If you're having difficulty (some specialists are booked months in advance), try sending him an email.

How to Find a Doctor's Email Address

"This is a true story," says Dr. Indu Subaiya, the co-founder of a health-care forum called Health 2.0. "A friend of mine needed to get his wife in to see a doctor for back pain. All the secretaries told them it would be weeks before they could get an appointment. They found the email address of one doctor who seemed like a good fit and wrote him a personal note explaining the urgency. He responded at 11 P.M., and she was in to see him the first thing in the morning the next day."

Here are some ways to find a doctor's email address:

1. Google the doctor. An email address might just pop up.
2. If the doctor works at a university or a hospital, see if the email address is listed on the university's website.
3. If the doctor's email address isn't there, look at how other names on the university's or hospital's website are listed, such as john.smith@university.edu or jsmith@hospital.com, and try the doctor's name using that format.

4. Use Google Scholar to see if the doctor has written any articles in medical journals. The author's email address is usually listed in these articles.

Once you have an appointment, the waiting isn't necessarily over. In fact, it may have just begun, as you might find yourself spending hours in the waiting room. A Las Vegas man named Aristotelis Belavilas waited for nearly four hours to see his doctor, and actually sued the doctor, winning $250 in small-claims court. If you're not quite that litigious, here are some other ideas for shortening the wait at the doctor's office. First, be a smart scheduler. Sean Kelley, a blogger for *Health* magazine, has diabetes and spends more than his fair share of time in doctors' waiting rooms. He suggests booking the first appointment in the morning, or the first appointment after lunch, and asking the scheduler to get you in on the lightest day of the week. If your doctor sees kids, Kelley says to avoid making an appointment on school holidays, when the schedule will be thick with kids. Once you're in the waiting room, speak up sooner rather than later if the doctor doesn't take you on time. "After fifteen minutes, max, ask the receptionist what's happening and if you've been forgotten," recommends Dr. L. Gordon Moore, who heads the Ideal Medical Practices Project, which aims to improve service and quality in doctors' offices.

If these tactics don't work and you still find yourself waiting aeons in the doctor's office, you might need to step it up a notch. Joanna Lipari, a psychologist in Southern California, once staged a waiting-room coup. "I ended up waiting two hours to see my gynecologist once, and I just went nuts," Lipari recalls. "I'm a New York Italian, and we don't go in for this kind of stuff. I was so irritated that I gathered together the other eight ladies in the room and joked, 'Let's stage a revolt.' " But that's exactly what they did. Each woman wrote a letter expressing frustration with the long waits. "I told her she's a wonderful doctor, but this really wasn't cool. I told her waiting so long was inconvenient, uncomfortable, and spoke badly for an otherwise exceptional medical practice," Lipari says. "I was trying to change her behavior, and it worked. They changed the way they scheduled appointments."

If long waits persist despite smart scheduling and complaints, you might need to think about finding a new doctor. If you go to the website for the Ideal Medical Practices Project (idealhealthnetwork .com), you'll see a list of physicians who have signed a pledge to work toward being on time for their patients. There is one more option when your doctor keeps you waiting: you can shut up and wait. During my third pregnancy, I had several ridiculously long waits for my obstetrician, and learned to bring a good book and my laptop to stay busy. Other people I know would have refused to see a doctor who subjected them to such long waits, but I liked this obstetrician. It helped that the nurses brought in bottles of water and granola bars to calm the wrath of all us hungry, pregnant women. Smart move.

Once you do get in to see the doctor, you might discover that he's rushed and harried. This is more than just annoying, as a rushed doctor is likely to make mistakes. But doctors are under such pressure today to crank out office visits that sometimes you really have to slow them down. For advice on this, I spoke with Larry Mauksch, a counselor and educator at the University of Washington Department of Family Medicine, who's been helping doctors communicate more successfully with patients for more than thirty years. First, Mauksch advises you to be aware of the doctor's behavior from the moment he enters the examining room. If the doctor launches into your problem without so much as a simple "Nice to see you" or "How's the family?," that's a red flag. "If a physician jumps immediately into addressing a problem before making a connection, patients should view this as a warning sign that the physician may feel hurried," Mauksch says. "Physicians who take even ten to twenty seconds to make a nonmedical connection are more likely to engage their patients in a productive partnership." He told me if your physician doesn't greet you it's time to slow him down. "When a physician forgets to make a connection, patients can say, 'How are you doing?' or 'You seem to be having a busy day,' and this may remind the physician to slow down."

Another way to get rid of that rushed-appointment feeling is to address fewer issues in one appointment (although of course if all your issues are urgent you don't have that luxury). Here's what Mauksch suggests: state all your medical concerns up front, even writing them down on a piece of paper and handing the list to the doctor. "The thoughtful physician will quickly determine if it is realistic or not to address all the problems in one visit," Mauksch says. "Patients should prioritize their lists and remember that sometimes spending more time on one to three concerns may be a better use of time than trying to address four or more problems on one day."

While you're in the middle of your appointment, Mauksch has more ideas about how to slow down a Dr. Speedy Gonzalez. He suggests saying something like "I have some questions or concerns that I wanted to run by you. Can I take a couple of minutes and tell you about them?" or "I need you to know what this has been like for me." If during the physical exam the doctor quickly writes down his findings without talking to you, ask him directly for his thoughts, with a query such as "Did you see any problems with my eardrum?" or "How do my heart and lungs sound?"

By the way, don't think that just because your doctor hands you a prescription you've had a well-thought-out appointment with a positive result. Dr. Deepak Chopra gave me one of the most important pieces of insider information about doctors I've ever heard. He told me that sometimes doctors just write a prescription to be done with a patient and move on to the next one. "They want to get patients in and out in five minutes, and it's so much easier to just write a prescription than to explain to the patient what's going on." But you absolutely need that explanation, and if you don't have it by the end of your appointment ask the doctor to listen while you repeat the plan back to him. (Say something like "Doctor, I understand I need to take an antibiotic for ten days and call you back in two days if I'm still feeling ill.") Actually, it's probably a good idea to do this even if you do understand your treatment plan, because you may only *think* you understand it. "If some aspect of the plan does not make sense, or is not feasible or attractive, this would be the time to tell the physician," Mauksch advises, noting that you can also ask the doctor to write down instructions for you. Repeating the plan back to the doctor, and having him confirm that you've understood, is a great way to fill in the "U" in your DUN form—the "understand the plan to get you better" section.

If you notice during your appointment that your doctor is more than just rushed, that he actually doesn't seem to be paying attention, take note. "Some doctors are regularly preoccupied and show this with poor eye contact, being fidgety, tapping their feet, or multitasking all the time," Mauksch says. "If this is a pattern across multiple visits and it's bothersome, it may be wise to look for a new doctor."

CONCLUSION: THE $500 DOCTOR'S APPOINTMENT

Sometimes I think we would all get more out of our eighteen minutes with the doctor if we were paying through the nose for it. If every doctor's appointment cost $500, you wouldn't just walk in and expect the doctor to have the answers; you would do everything in your power to make sure you came out of that appointment with solid, actionable pieces of advice. So the next time you go to the doctor, pretend that it's costing you a fortune. It will probably make you better prepared and prompt you to ask better questions. After all, nobody wants to pay $500 and walk out of a doctor's appointment saying "Huh?"

Final Checklist: How to Make Sure You Don't Walk Out of a Doctor's Appointment Saying "Huh?"

1. **Know what you're up against.** It's a challenge to accomplish anything meaningful in eighteen minutes with an interruption after the first twenty-three seconds, so you've got your work cut out for you.

2. **Be prepared for your appointment.** Write down your top three concerns, a list of questions for the doctor, a list of the medications you're taking, and your medical history if it's complicated.

3. **Bring in important documents.** Bring in test results from other doctors and imaging reports (MRIs, CT scans, etc.).

4. **Bring in a "Get It DUN!" worksheet.** You need to know your diagnosis, understand the plan to get you better, and know the next steps. (See page 180 in the appendix for a form.)

5. **Learn how to get an appointment on short notice.** When the secretary says the doctor is booked for the next six months, learn the tricks to getting in earlier, such as asking to speak with a nurse or an office manager, or emailing the doctor directly.

6. **Learn how to avoid long waits in the waiting room.** Book the first appointment in the morning or the first appointment after lunch. If your doctor sees children, avoid school holidays.

7. **Slow down a rushed doctor.** Certain phrases, such as "It seems like you're having a busy day" or "Can I take a couple of minutes to run some questions by you?" can slow down a harried physician.

8. **Ask your doctor for his email address.** Email addresses aren't useful only for getting an appointment on short notice; there's nothing like email for getting clarification after an ap-

pointment. You'll avoid the dreaded game of phone tag, and the instructions will be there for you in writing. More and more doctors are giving out email addresses these days; if your doctor won't do it, I wouldn't consider that a deal-breaker, but you might want to consider getting a new doctor.

9. **Take an advocate to your appointment.** Studies show that patients do better when they have a family member or a friend there to help ask questions and listen to the doctor's instructions.

10. **Repeat to yourself, "I'm paying $500 for this appointment."** Thinking this will force you to make the most of your time with your doctor. After all, you wouldn't walk out of the doctor's office with unanswered questions if you were paying a lot of money; you'd want to get your money's worth and avoid having to pay another $500 to get your questions answered at another appointment.

CHAPTER FOUR

How to Avoid a Misdiagnosis

Imagine waking up one day to find a lump the size of a golf ball sticking out of your side. That's what happened to Trisha Torrey, a fifty-two-year-old marketing executive in New York. Trisha showed the lump to her family physician, who immediately sent her to a surgeon. That very afternoon, the surgeon removed the lump, saying he'd call soon with the pathology results, which would reveal whether the lump was malignant or benign.

Cancer. That was the answer Trisha got two weeks later—cancer. And not just any kind of cancer but a rare blood cancer with a horrifying name: subcutaneous panniculitis-like T-cell lymphoma. Once Trisha had recovered from the initial shock of the terrifying diagnosis, she got on the Internet. "What I learned was that everyone died. And died fast," she wrote. "The longest anyone with SPTCL seemed to live was a couple of years, regardless of whether they received any treatment. And here I was with that disease—and scared to death."

At an appointment with her oncologist, Trisha asked the doctor for a ray of hope, for some possibility that she didn't really have cancer. Not a chance, the oncologist told her—not just one but two labs had made the diagnosis of subcutaneous panniculitis-like T-cell lymphoma. He ordered her to start chemotherapy—and fast. "You have no choice," the doctor told her. "Your lymphoma is highly aggressive, and if we don't start treatment we'll be measuring your life in months, not years." That August day, Trisha asked precisely how much time she had left to live if she didn't have the chemo. Without chemo, the doctor told her, she'd be dead before Christmas. Even with chemo, her prognosis wasn't good. A study at the Mayo Clinic of patients with SPTCL showed that even with treatment the average survival time was fifteen months.

Trisha feared that she was about to die. But was she?

MARCI AND THE BIG "OOPS"

The first time I met Marci Smith—our husbands went to school together at Georgia Tech—we talked for two hours nonstop. Marci epitomizes the word "life"—she glows with love for her husband, Tim, and their five-year-old son, Joshua. She nursed her mother through breast cancer, and when a teenager in her family needed help, she took him in and raised him as if he were her own. A sign-language interpreter, Marci works with deaf people in hospitals and courtrooms in Tennessee, where she and Tim and Joshua live, and where they love to hike in the Smoky Mountains.

Marci can remember the exact moment this full life came to a crashing halt. On February 9, 2007, at precisely 4:45 P.M., Marci's doctor called to tell her she had a brain tumor. He scheduled surgery to have the tumor removed, after which they'd do a biopsy to see whether it was benign or malignant. Marci had the surgery five days later, and Tim gave her a diamond anniversary ring, not knowing if it would be their last Valentine's Day together.

For several days, Marci and Tim waited anxiously to get the pathology results back. When the neurosurgeon called, he didn't immediately say whether the tumor was benign or malignant. Instead, he told Marci to go get a pencil. "Then he spelled it out for me, 'L-E-I-O-M-Y-O-S-A-R-C-O-M-A,' " Marci recalls. " 'That sounds like cancer,' I told him, and he said 'Yes.' " Like Trisha Torrey's disease, leiomyosarcoma is a rare and particularly aggressive form of cancer with a high death rate. According to one study, the *longest* anyone has lived with a "lymo" that starts in the brain is about two and a half years, and some people die within months of being diagnosed. Stunned, Marci set up an appointment to start chemotherapy the following week.

But she never kept that appointment.

For the next week, Marci lived on the Internet, becoming a lymo detective. She started with Google searches, using the information she'd learned from her neurosurgeon: she had a 2.5-millimeter leiomyosarcoma tumor on the left side of her head on the dura, a membrane that covers the brain. A full-body scan showed that she didn't have cancer anywhere else. Google led her to cancer websites, which in turn led her to articles in medical journals. Slowly, Marci learned that she not only had an extremely rare cancer, she had an extremely rare form of an extremely rare cancer. When a leiomyosarcoma is in the brain, it usually started somewhere else and spread to the brain. But Marci was told that she didn't have cancer anywhere else in her body, so the lymo must have started in her brain. Lymos that originate in the brain are so unusual that when they do occur doctors write them up in medical journals. As Marci read more on the Internet, she became puzzled. Everyone she read about who had a leiomyosarcoma that started in the brain had an immune problem, like AIDS, to begin with, or had had radiation earlier in life. Marci didn't have an immune disease, and she'd never had radiation.

Something didn't quite fit, so the day before she was supposed to start her first round of chemotherapy, Marci called and canceled the appointment. Her oncologist was horrified. Here was a woman with an aggressive cancer that could kill her within months and she was choosing not to get treatment. What was wrong with her? But Marci knew exactly what she was doing. Instead of going for the chemo appointment, she and her husband flew to Florida, where they had found a cancer center that specializes in sarcomas. The doctors there reviewed her records and tested a piece of her tumor. They told Marci that she didn't have leiomyosarcoma. Instead, they said, the tests showed that she had a glioblastoma multiforme, or GBM, the most common malignant brain tumor among adults.

Confused by the conflicting diagnoses, Marci asked her original neurosurgeon to send specimens of her tumor to two different laboratories. They both came back agreeing with the Florida doctors: she didn't have a lymo; she had the more common GBM. Her doctor then asked the first lab—the one that originally came up with the lymo diagnosis—to redo the test. The pathologist did, and delivered the news unapologetically. "Yes, we're wrong," they told Marci's neurosurgeon. "Upon further testing, we think it's a GBM." While it's a very serious diagnosis, a GBM is much more treatable than a lymo that starts in the brain.

What would have happened if Marci hadn't done her own detective work? She would probably be dead today. It's unlikely that chemo for a lymo would have done anything to combat her GBM, because the two diseases require different treatments. Marci is alive more than two years after doctors found the tumor only because she trusted that niggling little voice inside her that said, "I'm no doctor, but something about this diagnosis just doesn't sound right."

WHAT THE STUDIES SAY

Studies show it's not a matter of if but when a misdiagnosis will happen to you. No one knows the exact percentage of diagnoses that turn out to be wrong, but several studies put the figure at around 10 to 15 percent, with at least one study putting it as high as 25 percent. If you take the low end, this means that one out of every ten diagnoses you receive from a doctor will be wrong. At the high end, one out of four diagnoses will be wrong. Either way, it appears that at some point in your life you'll be on the receiving end of a misdiagnosis.

Sometimes a misdiagnosis is the fault of the doctor who examined you, but often it's because of a doctor you've never met. For example, as Marci found out, pathologists, the doctors who look at tissue samples under a microscope, make mistakes. In one study, pathologists were presented with tissue samples and asked to decide if they were normal, cancerous, or precancerous. It turns out that the pathologist made the wrong call in close to 12 percent of the specimens. Another class of physicians you'll never meet, but who could play a crucial role in your care, are radiologists, the doctors who read X-rays, MRIs, and other images. To test the accuracy of radiologists' readings, researchers at Michigan State University showed sixty chest X-rays to one hundred radiologists. When the radiologists were asked "Is this X-ray normal?," they disagreed with one another 20 percent of the time, which, by definition, means that some of them had to be wrong. When a single radiologist reread the same sixty X-rays at a later time, he contradicted his earlier analysis from 5 to 10 percent of the time.

A misdiagnosis can also be the fault of the lab test itself. At the height of the swine-flu outbreak in the fall of 2009, I did a story about a sick nine-year-old girl who went to the emergency room two days in a row and took a flu test; both times, the test said she didn't have the flu and the doctor sent her home. On the third day, when the child was so weak she couldn't walk, her mother carried her into the hospital, and she spent the next six weeks in the intensive-care unit and nearly died. Further testing showed that she'd had swine flu—also called H1N1 flu—the entire time. I then learned from infectious-disease experts that the flu test she took, which is routinely given in ERs and doctor's offices across the country, is wrong *about half the time.*

I also remember that when I was pregnant with my first daughter and ill I took a urine test. My obstetrician took one look at the results and stabbed the paper with his index finger, saying, "If this number was right, you'd be dead." (Obviously, this was a mistake, but other types of goofs in a urine or blood test could lead the doctor down the wrong path.) There's yet another way that a misdiagnosis can happen. A pathologist's or radiologist's report could be right, but your own doctor could read it incorrectly or misinterpret it. That's what happened to Doug Smith, who identified his own cancer. (You can read his story on page 65.)

Sometimes a misdiagnosis is rooted in a housekeeping mistake. Researchers at the University of Chicago surveyed eight family-medicine practices and found that in an eight-month period there were *966 testing-process errors.* All sorts of things went wrong. Sometimes the doctor's office ordered the wrong tests; at other times the results were never reported by the lab, or the results weren't placed in the patient's chart.

This isn't terribly surprising given the disorganization in many medical offices. One doctor has given us a detailed—and frightening—description of how his office operates. "A doctor's office is always on the brink of chaos—with an incredible amount of information coming in and going out, a large number of phone calls, insurance-company headaches, and personnel situations that can throw the best system flat on its face," says Dr. Robert Lamberts, a family doctor from Augusta, Georgia, and a popular blogger. "I order hundreds of tests every week. I just cannot keep track of them all. Some test results will get sent to the wrong doctor, and some never get sent at all. Despite our best efforts to develop a system that will close this loop, there are some documents I just don't get."

"There are some documents I just don't get"? Yikes! This isn't what we patients want to hear! You know what happens if your doctor doesn't receive a crucial test result? You got it—it greatly increases the odds that he'll arrive at the wrong diagnosis.

Given the sometimes deadly ramifications of a misdiagnosis, you would think doctors and hospitals would do everything they could to avoid making this kind of error. Sadly, that's not always the case. "Diagnostic errors are simply not a priority for health care organizations," Dr. Mark Graber wrote in the *Journal on Quality and Patient Safety.* One reason for this, Dr. Graber goes on to say, is that doctors often deny that the problem even exists. "Physicians responsible for making medical decisions seldom perceive their own error rates as problematic," he writes. Some of the foremost experts on misdiagnoses, such as Dr. Graber, who is chief of the medical service at the Veterans Affairs Medical Center in Northport, New York, and Dr. Pat Croskerry, a professor of emergency medicine and medical education at Dalhousie University in Halifax, Canada, have tried for years to get hospitals and doctors to decrease misdiagnoses by using checklists, better communication, and improvements in medical education. But so far many of these suggestions haven't been adopted. Doctors don't even talk all that much about misdiagnoses, let alone implement systems to decrease their frequency. "Diagnosing is the most important thing a doctor does," Dr. Croskerry told me. "It's the very essence of a doctor's being. Yet the first conference on misdiagnoses was held just last year! That's remarkable."

The Man Who Caught His Own Cancer

When Doug Smith felt some discomfort in his chest, his primary-care physician, Dr. Jim Jirjis, immediately ordered tests, including a CT scan. After the scan, Dr. Jirjis was happy to learn from the radiologist that Smith's heart was just fine. "I was relieved and immediately called him on the telephone and said, 'Great news,' " says Dr. Jirjis, an internist at Vanderbilt University Medical Center in Nashville, Tennessee.

Dr. Jirjis figured that was it—the report showed that Doug was just fine. But Doug didn't let it end there, and thank goodness he didn't. He went to his computer and read the radiologist's actual CT-scan report online. (Unlike most of us, Doug's medical records are electronic.) As he read, Doug noticed this single sentence deep into the report about something the radiologist noticed on his thyroid: "12 mm low-density right thyroid lobe lesion is technically indeterminate. Correlation with sonography is suggested." Now, Doug is no doctor—he's a chief financial officer for a local company in Nashville—but he's smart enough to know that the word "lesion" isn't good (it was large enough to measure), and that the phrase "sonography is suggested" meant that the radiologist was trying to tell Dr. Jirjis that more needed to be done, that there was a next step to be taken.

That lesion on his thyroid turned out to be cancer. Because he double-checked his doctor, Doug caught his cancer early enough for it to be easily treated. Dr. Jirjis isn't happy that he missed the reference to the thyroid lesion, but he isn't surprised, either. "Most physicians are reviewing an enormous amount of lab results every day," he told me. "The patient is reviewing just one person's lab results." Lesson learned: try to read the results of your tests and imaging reports. You don't have to be a doctor to understand them.

SOLUTIONS: HELPING YOUR DOCTOR
GET YOUR DIAGNOSIS RIGHT

There are several steps you can take to help your doctor make the right diagnosis. Before I explain them, I'd like to introduce you to a few of my "diagnostic heroes."

MY "DIAGNOSTIC HEROES"

Marci and Trisha are two of my diagnostic heroes, and I've written about several others in my "Empowered Patient" column, including Brad Burns, an auto-insurance adjuster from Oklahoma, who caught a misdiagnosis in his elderly mother. Nancy Burns had complained one day that her shoulder was hurting. "I told her to go to the doctor, and she came back and said, 'The doctor says I tore my rotator cuff. I'm starting physical therapy next week.' "

Brad's no doctor, but he has a lot of common sense, and this rotator-cuff diagnosis sounded, well, weird. Brad knew that rotator-cuff injuries tend to happen to baseball pitchers and other people who spend a lot of time raising their arms above their shoulders. His sixty-six-year-old mother stayed at home and hardly did any activity at all. Brad took his mother to another doctor for a second opinion. This doctor did a scan of her shoulder and found something that looked troubling. He then did another scan and, as Brad put it, "her whole body lit up" with cancer. Nancy Burns didn't have a torn rotator cuff; she had cancer in her shoulder and throughout her body. She died a few months later. In her case, it wouldn't have made much of a difference if the diagnosis had been right from the start because her cancer was so advanced, but Brad's story points to a bigger truth: when we get a hunch—a feeling that something just doesn't sound right—we're often right, even if we have no medical training.

High School Girl Diagnoses Her Own Disease in Science Class

For eight years, Jessica Terry, a high school senior, suffered from stomach pain so horrible that it brought her to her knees. Her doctors couldn't figure out the cause, but one day Jessica figured it out on her own—in her science class.

In her advanced-placement class, Jessica was looking under the microscope at slides of her own intestinal tissue—slides her pathologist had said were completely normal—and she spotted an area of inflamed tissue called a granuloma, a clear indication that she had Crohn's disease.

"It's weird I had to solve my own medical problem," Jessica told her local TV station. "There were just no answers anywhere. . . . I was always sick."

"She was pretty excited about finding the granuloma," Mary-Margaret Welch, Jessica's teacher in Sammamish, Washington, recalls. "She said, 'Ms. Welch! Ms. Welch! Come over here. I think I've got something!' "

"I said, 'Jeez, it certainly looks like one to me,' " Welch said. "I snapped a picture of it on the microscope and emailed it to the pathologist. Within twenty-four hours he sent back an email saying yes, this is a granuloma."

Pathologists also sometimes miss important findings for other diseases, Dr. Mark Graber says. "This story carries a valuable lesson about how errors are found," he told me. "It's very often by 'fresh eyes,' just like in Jessica's case. Some specialty centers, recognizing the reality of perceptual error and the power of a second independent reading, are now requiring second reviews on certain types of smears and pathology specimens."

My other diagnostic hero is Trisha Torrey. When we left Trisha earlier in this chapter, she was on the verge of starting chemotherapy for subcutaneous panniculitis-like T-cell lymphoma (or SPTCL), a rare and highly aggressive form of blood cancer. Like Marci, Trisha went on the Internet not to disprove her doctors but to learn more about her disease, and, like Marci, she noticed something strange when she began reading about the symptoms of SPTCL. "I learned . . . I should have symptoms I didn't have—like fever, lethargy, and weight loss. I had plenty of energy to play golf once or twice a week. Physically, I felt just fine," she told me. When she brought this discrepancy to her doctor's attention, he pointed out that she did have two symptoms of the lymphoma, night sweats and hot flashes. But wait a second, Trisha thought to herself, I'm a fifty-two-year-old woman. Aren't night sweats and hot flashes also signs of menopause? She asked her oncologist if there was any possibility the diagnosis was wrong. He said absolutely not, since not one but two labs had confirmed it.

There was mounting pressure for Trisha to start chemotherapy, and her doctors asked her what in the world she was waiting for. What she was waiting for was a second opinion, but she didn't know whom to go to, and since she had "lousy" insurance she didn't have the money to go from doctor to doctor in the hope of finding a smart one.

In the end, what saved Trisha Torrey was a few glasses of wine.

Trisha had pretty much kept mum about her deadly diagnosis until one night when she was having dinner with friends and wine loosened her tongue. She told them about her deadly diagnosis, and one of her friends, once she got over the initial shock, suggested that Trisha see an oncologist friend of hers. Trisha called to set up the appointment, and it turned out this doctor had experience treating SPTCL. Trisha called the office of her original oncologist and asked that her medical records be sent to her. In the days spent waiting for her appointment with this second doctor, Trisha read through her records and she couldn't believe her eyes. The labs *hadn't* said that she had SPTCL, as the first doctor had told her. They said something quite different. One lab report indicated that the tumor was "most suspicious for" SPTCL, and the second lab report stated it was "most consistent with" SPTCL. That's hardly definitive! As Trisha read on, she grew even more suspicious. The pathologist who wrote the second lab report said he'd sent a sample of the tumor to a third lab for additional testing. She searched furiously through her medical files and found no results from this third lab. She asked her original oncologist for the results from the third lab, and at first he couldn't find them. Eventually, with Trisha's prodding, he did. The verdict: the results from this third lab showed that the tumor was benign.

Armed with this new information, Trisha saw the oncologist her friend had recommended, and he sent a sample of her tumor to a lab at the National Institutes of Health. Three weeks later, she received confirmation that her lump was harmless. Trisha wasn't about to die. She didn't have cancer. If she hadn't done her Internet research, Trisha would have been on the receiving end of highly toxic chemotherapy that she absolutely didn't need. Today, Trisha shares the wisdom she gained from her experience with others as the leader for about.com's patient-empowerment site and in her book *You Bet Your Life.*

So what solutions can we learn from these diagnostic heroes? First, we should learn we need to get out of our fog and recognize the harsh reality that misdiagnoses happen with some frequency. This can be tough to do, because it means acknowledging that when you're at your weakest point, when your very life depends on the guy or gal in the white coat, the person helping you is fallible and might mess things up. "Many times diseases mask themselves as other diseases, so you're completely fooled," Dr. Jerome Kassirer, a former editor-in-chief of *The New England Journal of Medicine,* explained to me. "And tests are imperfect. There are false positives and false negatives, and you get fooled all the time. Patients don't fully appreciate that."

Despite all the fancy scans and the blood tests and the whiz-bang technology, there's much uncertainty in medicine. "Most people aren't aware of how imperfect a science medicine really is," Dr. Croskerry says. Then he paused for a moment. "Actually, medicine's not a science at all. It's a practice. It's a skill and a craft. But it's definitely not a science." Then he said something that made *me* pause. "Patients are much more vulnerable than they know."

Only after you realize your own vulnerability can you take action to catch a misdiagnosis. Once you recognize that doctors and tests aren't perfect, you'll know to pay attention to your hunches as Brad did and, if something sounds weird (a rotator cuff on a sixty-six-year-old woman who sits around all day?), to trust that impulse. You should also do what Trisha did and research your diagnosis on the Internet, and, like Doug, you should read crucial test results yourself. (Don't be intimidated; Doug isn't a medical professional, and he was able to understand his CT-scan report.) You should also remember to call your doctor if you haven't been given your test results in a timely fashion. "No news is not good news," says Dr. Saul Weingart, the vice president for patient safety at the Dana-Farber Cancer Institute. "It might be that the report fell down behind someone's desk." You should also learn to ask the one question that could save your life.

Five Red Flags That You've Been Misdiagnosed

1. You go online and discover that your symptoms don't match your diagnosis.
2. Your diagnosis is based on one test.
3. Your symptoms are common, and your diagnosis isn't.
4. You don't get better with treatment.
5. Your symptoms are consistent with several diseases, and your doctor can't explain to you how she picked one from the list.

THE QUESTION THAT COULD SAVE YOUR LIFE

With one simple question, you could save yourself from a misdiagnosis. The question is stunningly simple. Here it is: "Doctor, what else could this be?"

Yes, that's it—six words that could put your doctor on the path to getting it right. Dr. Jerome Groopman made this question famous in his book *How Doctors Think*. He explained that doctors sometimes have a tendency to do what's called "anchoring," and it's bad. "Anchoring is a shortcut in thinking where a person doesn't consider multiple possibilities but quickly and firmly latches on to a single one, sure that he has thrown his anchor down just where he needs to be," he writes. This is an eloquent way of saying it's human nature to have a hard time changing your mind when you've made a judgment about something. For a doctor, this means sticking with a diagnosis even when she should consider other possibilities. Asking that magic question—"Doctor, what else could this be?"—could help your doctor open her eyes to other possible diagnoses.

As an example, let's use Barbara Robbins and her daughter Stephanie, whom we met in chapter 1. For ten years, every time Stephanie ate, she suffered from bloody diarrhea and terrible stomach cramps. When Barbara first took Stephanie to the gastroenterologist, at the age of thirteen, the doctor diagnosed irritable bowel syndrome. It took ten years—and another doctor—to get the right diagnosis, which was ulcerative colitis. During that time, Stephanie's weight dropped to 113 pounds—and she's six feet tall. Once she was treated for ulcerative colitis, Stephanie recovered, gained weight, and thrived.

Did Stephanie need to suffer for ten years, or could Barbara have done something to catch that misdiagnosis earlier? There's a chance Barbara could have saved her daughter many years of pain with that million-dollar question: "Doctor, what else could this be?" This one question could have cued the original doctor into listing other possible reasons for Stephanie's cramps, diarrhea, and weight loss.

I asked Dr. Corey Siegel, the director of the Inflammatory Bowel Disease Center at Dartmouth-Hitchcock Medical Center in New Hampshire, to explain what else besides IBS could have been causing Stephanie's problems. He told me several diseases could have been at the root of her symptoms: everything from a bacterial infection to lactose intolerance to a parasite. Dr. Siegel, a great believer in shared decision-making between patients and doctors, told me that armed with that list of possibilities it would have been very reasonable for Barbara to ask why, given such a large number of possibilities, the doctor arrived at the diagnosis of irritable bowel syndrome. After hearing his answer, Barbara could then have asked another question: "I understand you think IBS is the reason for her problems. Since you just told me there are many other diseases that can cause these symptoms, are there any tests that would help us sort this out, and do you think my daughter should have them?" By asking this question, Dr. Siegel says, Barbara would have learned that a colonoscopy could have diagnosed the ulcerative colitis.

Of course, there's a strong possibility this doctor was so "anchored" in his IBS diagnosis that he would have blown off Barbara's questions altogether, insisting at every turn that he was 100 percent sure Stephanie had IBS. In that case, Barbara could have gone on the Internet and clearly seen with a simple Google search that many diseases can cause diarrhea, cramping, and weight loss. This would have been her cue that this doctor had faulty thinking and she needed a second opinion. One note here about getting second opinions: if you can, get one from someone who's not connected to the first doctor (meaning they work in different practices, universities, etc.). Physicians are only human, and might have a hard time saying their buddy (or someone who sends a lot of business their way) got it wrong.

HOW TO HELP YOUR DOCTOR GET IT RIGHT

In chapter 3, we talked about how to have a successful doctor's appointment, but, more specifically, let's discuss what you can do in the doctor's office to avoid a misdiagnosis. In addition to asking, "Doctor, what else could this be?" you need to make sure you're explaining your symptoms and health history the right way, since your explanation of your illness will greatly influence your doctor's thinking. In fact, your personal story is just as important as, some-times even more important than, a blood-test result or an MRI. Told well, your personal story can lead your doctor down the right cognitive path to figuring out what ails you. Told poorly, your story can confuse him and distract him, leading him to make the wrong diagnosis. Your explanation of what's wrong can truly make or break a diagnosis, and doctors tell me that too often they get ram-bling stories like this: "I've been having sharp pains in my elbow and I don't know when it started, but it might have been when I was visiting my grandmother for Thanksgiving and I hit my elbow on the corner of the dining-room table while I was reaching for the sweet-potato soufflé, but then again maybe it was when I was play-ing doubles tennis and hit a strong backhand and I couldn't stop playing even though I was in pain because I didn't want to disap-point my partner."

Your story should be more focused. When did your problem start? Have your symptoms improved over time, or have they got-ten worse? What treatments have you already tried? Did they make you feel better or worse? Remember to be specific. "When you say you're tired, what does 'tired' mean?" asks Dr. Kassirer. "Does it mean you can't stand up from a chair? You can't drive a car? Or does it mean you're just sleepier than usual? The more specific patients can be about their symptoms, the better it is for the doctor." Also, know your medical history: what you've been diagnosed with in the past and what drugs, treatments, and surgeries you've had. Next, know your family history. If you aren't sure whether Grandma had Huntington's disease or Hodgkin's disease, ask your mother before you go to see the doctor. These details matter, and it's your respon-sibility to know them; showing up poorly informed only hurts you. Also, when you have a doctor's appointment, bring in documents from other offices, such as lab results, imaging reports, and physi-cians' notes. Take them to your doctor yourself; getting the other doctor to forward these things could require an act of Congress.

Before you leave the doctor's office, write down your diagnosis and other details on a "Get It DUN!" worksheet, which you'll find on page 180 of the appendix. Spelling counts—you want to be able to Google your diagnosis when you get home, and whether you have hypothyroidism or hyperthyroidism matters a great deal. (For more information on how to research your diagnosis on the Internet, see chapter 5.) When you do sit down to Google, the first thing you'll want to do is make sure your diagnosis exists. Sounds crazy, right? How could your doctor diagnose you with a nonexistent illness? Well, it happens. In fact, I know of a doctor who diagnosed *another doctor* with a made-up disease. I guess this doctor was hoping his patient wouldn't notice, but indeed he did, because the patient was Dr. Groopman. In *How Doctors Think,* Dr. Groopman describes his struggles over the years with wrist pain. Even something as simple as opening a bottle of juice resulted in excruciating pain erupting in his right wrist. At times he couldn't even move his hand. Just holding a mug of coffee became painful, writing a few sentences with a pen caused his hand to swell up, and typing became impossible.

Dr. Groopman went to a hand surgeon he calls Dr. A, who was well known in Boston's medical community for treating the injuries of professional athletes. Dr. Groopman had several follow-up visits with Dr. A, and each time the hand surgeon tried something else—he put the wrist in a splint, tested Dr. Groopman for arthritis, gave him a steroid injection in the wrist—but nothing provided more than temporary relief. Then, about a year after his initial visit, Dr. A announced that he thought Dr. Groopman had a "hyperactive synovium" and suggested surgery to fix it. Hmm, Dr. Groopman thought to himself, I'm no specialist in diseases of the bones and joints, but I've never heard of a hyperactive synovium. He consulted another hand surgeon, who hadn't heard of it, either. Dr. Groopman's conclusion: after a frustrating year of failing to nail down exactly what was wrong, Dr. A "invented something to respond to my plaintive questioning and suggested an operation that could be damaging."

Lesson learned: if a doctor can throw a made-up diagnosis at another doctor, he can throw one at you, too, so do the due diligence and make sure your diagnosis actually exists. Then, move on to the next step: see if the symptoms you're having match up with the symptoms listed for your diagnosis on reliable websites. (To figure out whether a website is reliable, see the next chapter.) Performing this symptom check was Trisha Torrey's first step toward realizing that she'd been misdiagnosed, since the check revealed that she didn't have most of the symptoms of the lymphoma. Another way to detect a misdiagnosis is to find out which medical tests are usually done to arrive at your diagnosis and see if you've had them. Let's say, for example, you learn on the Internet that doctors usually do a certain blood test or X-ray to detect your disease. If you didn't have those tests, that's a red flag that you might not have the right diagnosis.

Should you suspect a misdiagnosis every time you go to the doctor? No. If your throat hurts and the doctor does a strep test that turns out positive, you probably don't need to spend hours on the Internet checking to see if it's really something else. However, there are certain situations where you should be wary of a misdiagnosis. For example, be on your toes when doctors pass information along to one another, since information can get lost pretty easily when it goes from one doctor to another. In an article aptly titled "Fumbled Handoffs: One Dropped Ball After Another," Dr. Tejal Ghandi, of Harvard Medical School, describes how a patient's diagnosis of tuberculosis was substantially delayed because of a lack of communication between doctors who worked in shifts at the hospital. Doctors failed to tell one another about crucial test results, and the patient died in the intensive-care unit. You don't have to be in the hospital for this to happen. Let's say, for example, that your doctor orders an important test, goes on vacation, and asks her partner to follow up on the results. If those two doctors don't communicate well, those test results could fall through the cracks and you could end up with a misdiagnosis. Do your best to remember what tests were ordered so you can remind your doctors if necessary.

Brad Burns—the man whose mother didn't really have a torn rotator cuff—learned the hard way that one of the most important ways you can prevent a misdiagnosis is to trust your intuition, that little voice that says something about your doctor's diagnosis isn't right. If something doesn't make sense, ask your doctor about it. If you don't understand her answers, keep asking until you do. If you still don't get it, remember that you're a smart person, and if something doesn't make sense to you there's a good chance it doesn't make sense at all. The diagnosis might be just plain wrong.

When your inner voice speaks to you, be relentless about pursuing its message. Robert Hanscom, a lawyer and a vice president for loss prevention and patient safety at Harvard's Risk Management Foundation, told me a chilling story about a young woman who complained of stomach and chest pains. Her doctor prescribed a medicine for gastric reflux. When this didn't work, a second doctor prescribed another drug for gastric reflux. This didn't work, either. It turned out that all this time the woman had acute pancreatitis, a potentially deadly inflammation of the pancreas. She went into kidney failure because of the misdiagnosis, and will probably be on dialysis for the rest of her life. When she sued the hospital, Hanscom read what she said at the legal proceedings and his heart sank. "In her deposition, she said nobody was listening to her, so she kind of gave up," Hanscom told me. "When I read that, I thought, Oh God, I wish you hadn't given up."

CONCLUSION

Doug Smith's physician, Dr. Jim Jirjis, doesn't hide the fact that he missed Doug's thyroid cancer. In fact, Dr. Jirjis invited me to Vanderbilt to do a story about how he missed—and how Doug found—the cancer. This was an amazingly brave thing for Dr. Jirjis to do, but I know not all physicians are like him. I've heard some doctors get downright testy when patients start challenging a diagnosis. If your doctor ever makes you feel bad for asking questions, here's what you should do: think of the prominent physicians—leaders in their field, editors of prestigious journals—who *encourage* patients to get more involved, who say that patients need to ask *more* questions, that a patient's involvement can be *the* key to getting the right diagnosis. I've heard this over and over from doctors. "Properly educated, patients are ideal partners to help reduce the likelihood of [diagnostic] errors," Dr. Graber wrote in *The American Journal of Medicine.* "They are perfectly positioned to prevent, detect, and mollify many system-based as well as cognitive factors that detract from timely and accurate diagnosis." Do your research, ask questions, and don't stop until you're satisfied you've received the right answers. "Your doctor may hate you for doing that, but it's your body," Dr. Kassirer told me.

So when you're sitting in the examining room, feeling intimidated about asking your doctor questions, say to yourself, "The former editor of *The New England Journal of Medicine,* who's a distinguished professor at Tufts University School of Medicine and a visiting professor at Stanford University School of Medicine, says I must do this!"

That should make you sit up a little straighter in your paper robe—and may help you avoid becoming the victim of a misdiagnosis.

Final Checklist: How to Avoid a Misdiagnosis

1. **At the doctor's office, tell your medical history well and take good notes.** Be specific and concise about what's bothering you. Write down important details on a "Get It DUN!"

worksheet. (See page 180 of the appendix.) Remember, spelling counts, as you'll want to Google your diagnosis later.

2. **Be the link between your physicians.** For safety's sake, assume your doctors don't talk to one another. If one doctor orders a test, get the results and take them in to your other doctor.

3. **Accept the fact that medicine is more of an art than a science.** When you receive your diagnosis, realize that it might be wrong. In most, but not all, cases, diagnosing a problem is a complex thought process for the doctor, with many opportunities for mistakes.

4. **Research your diagnosis on the Internet.** Make sure your disease actually exists. Make sure your symptoms match the disease you've been diagnosed as having. Check to see if there are any tests that are customarily done to arrive at your diagnosis. (For more information on how to do health research on the Internet, see chapter 5.)

5. **Be aware of the red flags of misdiagnosis.** As you do your research, ask yourself these questions: Is your diagnosis based on only one lab test? (If the test was wrong, your diagnosis is wrong.) Are your symptoms common (e.g., fatigue, a sore throat), but your diagnosis is rare? Have your symptoms not improved with treatment? If the answer to any of these questions is yes, it doesn't mean you've been misdiagnosed; it just means you should be especially wary.

6. **Trust your gut instincts.** If you feel your diagnosis is wrong, trust that feeling and don't ignore it. Be relentless about pursuing it; remember the woman who will probably be on dialysis for the rest of her life because she didn't follow through when she had the feeling her doctors were wrong.

7. **Ask, "Doctor, what else could this be?"** If you suspect a misdiagnosis—especially if you're not getting any better with the doctor's treatment—ask your doctor this million-dollar

question. It will help her think about constructing a list of other diseases that could be causing your symptoms.

8. **Ask your doctor why she chose this particular diagnosis.** If more than one diagnosis exists for your symptoms, ask your doctor why she singled out the one she did. Don't accept "Because that's what I think you have" as an answer. Ask her for the specific reasons that she thinks you have one disease instead of another.

9. **Ask if there are any tests that would help determine the right diagnosis.** If you haven't had these tests, ask why. Asking this question will help fine-tune your doctor's thought process.

10. **Seek a second opinion.** If you suspect a misdiagnosis, or if your questions aren't being answered, arrange to see another doctor. Try to go to a physician who isn't connected to your own doctor—friends might hesitate to contradict one another.

CHAPTER FIVE

How to Become an Internet MD (Medical Detective)

On the day after Christmas in 2001, the American Medical Association issued a press release encouraging all Americans to make ten New Year's resolutions. The nation's doctors urged us to eat better and exercise, get our cholesterol tested and our children immunized, and not to smoke or abuse drugs or alcohol. "These resolutions are simply a few of the things you can do to make positive, healthy lifestyle changes," wrote Dr. Richard F. Corlin, who was the president of the AMA at the time.

The nation's top doctors' group advised us to do one more thing to stay healthy. "Trust your physician, not a chat room," they said. People who go online, the AMA warned, "may be putting their lives at risk."

Apparently, the Internet is a scary place for America's doctors.

Although 2001 was many years ago, from what I can tell many doctors still consider the Internet terrifying territory, a place to tread not at all or only with great trepidation. I know I've been on the receiving end of some serious attitude when I've mentioned something I read online to a doctor, and many other patients have reported the same treatment. "One [of my doctors] commented that online information is like scribble on a bathroom wall," a patient commented in a report about online medical information. "[I guess he meant] trash or untrustworthy." Another patient said her neurologist "went wild with fury that I would *dare* look up my problems online." A third commented, "My child's GI [doctor] refused to even look at the information I brought in. . . . Most roll their eyes." Even Tara Parker-Pope, a reporter for *The New York Times* and one of the nation's most respected medical journalists, got a little eye roll herself from her mother's oncologist. "I asked him about new targeted therapies being studied for esophageal cancer," she said. "He shook his head in annoyance. 'I can tell someone has been spending time on the Internet,' he said dismissively."

In many ways, the Internet has become the great divide between doctors and patients. Nearly every patient uses the Internet in some way these days, but doctors seem to hate it more than they despise managed care, declining insurance reimbursements, or patients who stiff them on their bills. What your doctor won't tell you (maybe because he doesn't know) is that on the Internet you can learn about medical advances months, or even years, before *he* hears about them. What your doctor won't tell you is that on the Internet you can find solutions to your problems besides the ones he has told you about. What your doctor won't tell you is that the Internet can save your life.

Your doctor won't tell you how to harness the truly amazing health powers of the Internet. But I will.

MARIAN, KEN, AND FAY: THE NEWEST GENERATION OF INTERNET PATIENTS

The Internet truly has revolutionized what it means to be a patient. In fact, things were so different in the pre-Internet days that it's hard to remember what it was like, so let me remind you. Learning about your health was, to put it bluntly, a pain in the neck. Information was almost exclusively in the realm of health professionals, so anytime you had a health question, no matter how small, you had to call your doctor's office or get yourself to a library. Here's an account from the e-Patient Scholars Working Group, a coalition of physicians, patients, and advocates, about the lengths to which one man had to go in the pre-Internet days in order to get access to the health information he needed.

> One morning in 1994, the year Netscape released the first commercial Web browser, the Englewood Hospital library in Englewood, New Jersey, received a most unusual call. The caller identified himself as Dr. Harold Blakely, a local family practitioner. He gave the librarian a bibliographic citation for an article in a medical journal and asked her to make him a copy and leave it on the table outside the library door, where he could pick it up on his evening rounds. This request was not unusual. The hospital librarians frequently left copies of journal articles that local doctors could pick up after hours.
>
> Later that afternoon, the caller phoned again, checking to be sure that his article was ready. But the library's director, Kathy Lindner, took the call this time. Ms. Lindner knew Dr. Blakely. But she did not recognize the caller's voice. After a brief discussion with a colleague, she phoned Dr. Blakely's office. After several minutes a bewildered Dr. Blakely came to the phone. He assured Ms. Lindner that neither he nor anyone in his office had called the hospital library that day.
>
> Half an hour after the library closed that evening, a nervous, well-dressed man with carefully barbered gray hair entered the hospital through a side entrance. Walking with a cane, he passed the elevator, climbed the stairs with some difficulty, and continued down the second floor hallway toward the medical library. As he picked up the envelope with Dr. Blakely's name on it, a hospital security guard stepped out of the doorway where he had been waiting and asked him to identify himself.
>
> Under the questioning of the hospital's security service, he admitted that he was Edwin Murphy, a 58-year-old insurance

agent with a chronic hip problem. Dr. Blakely, his physician, had been urging him to undergo a promising new surgical procedure. Mr. Murphy was intrigued but not convinced. He wanted to know more about the potential risks and benefits of the proposed procedure and had repeatedly asked Dr. Blakely to help him obtain a copy of the definitive review article which had recently appeared in a major medical journal. In spite of his repeated requests, Dr. Blakely had not done so. Finally, in desperation, Mr. Murphy had decided that there was only one way to obtain this vital medical information he needed: he would have to impersonate his own physician.

Imagine if Mr. Murphy had needed this information in our day and age. He could have found the study he needed on the Internet in about fifteen minutes—and avoided a run-in with the law! I'm so grateful I live in the age of the Internet; I'm always astounded at what patients manage to do online. Just as in chapter 4 I told you about my "diagnostic heroes," here are my "Internet heroes": patients who used the Internet to get a diagnosis when their doctors had failed them, or found treatments on the Internet that their doctor had never told them about.

DARRAH SANDMAIER: You know what water sounds like when it's sloshing around in a pail? Sixteen-year-old Darrah Sandmaier heard this sound all the time, like a ringing in her ears, and in addition she had headaches and neck pain. Her mother, Marian, took her to the pediatrician's office and asked what he thought it was. "Hard to say," the pediatrician answered. "Call back in two weeks if she's having problems."

This didn't satisfy Marian, and, unlike the hapless Mr. Murphy, she had access to the Internet and knew how to use it. The next day, Marian remembered that Darrah had recently started taking an antibiotic for a skin problem, so she sat down at her computer and

Googled "minocycline" and "side effects." She quickly learned that in rare cases minocycline can cause pseudotumor cerebri, an accumulation of fluid around the brain that can lead to headaches, neck pain, and, yes, a sloshing sound inside your head. Marian told Darrah to stop taking the antibiotics, and she took her back to the dermatologist who had prescribed the minocycline. The doctor dismissed Marian's findings on the Internet, but nonetheless switched Darrah to a new antibiotic. When they got home, Marian checked the side effects of the new medication and found that it, too, could cause pseudotumor cerebri. Marian told the e-Patient Scholars Working Group:

> Two doctors had now shrugged their shoulders at my daughter's symptoms. . . . And through it all, our daughter's symptoms continued to worsen. Yet who was I to diagnose a rare disorder—on the Internet, no less? These two physicians had 30 years of clinical experience between them. All I had was a tall stack of Web printouts and a passion for my child's health.
>
> I called Darrah's dermatologist and pediatrician and told them that I had rejected their diagnoses. With the help of the Internet, I had made my own tentative diagnosis and would proceed accordingly. When I said the words *pseudotumor cerebri,* they both became very quiet.

The Sandmaiers took Darrah to a neuro-ophthalmologist at the University of Pennsylvania, saying nothing about their suspicions. After a lengthy battery of neurological tests, the specialist announced her verdict: Darrah had pseudotumor cerebri, which can damage the optic nerve, producing vision difficulties and, in severe cases, blindness. Thanks to her mother's quick work on the Internet, Darrah stopped taking the antibiotics early enough to prevent permanent damage. Her mother's "Internet diagnosis" probably saved her sight.

DR. KENNETH YOUNER: When Dr. Kenneth Youner, a gastroenterologist, found that his kidney cancer had spread to his chest, he went to his oncologist to map out a battle plan. During the discussion, his doctor recommended a drug called Sutent, and didn't mention any other possible treatments. But Ken had spent time on the Internet and was surprised that his oncologist hadn't mentioned Interleukin-2, another drug used for kidney cancer, which boosts the body's immune system to fight off, or even destroy, cancer cells.

Since his doctor never mentioned IL-2, Ken brought it up himself. The doctor dismissed it, pointing out that the drug can cause kidney damage, heart attacks, and in rare cases even death. In fact, the drug is so toxic that patients have to stay in the hospital while it's being administered.

What the oncologist didn't tell Ken—but what Ken knew because he'd been online—is that for some patients IL-2 is a wonder drug. In about 10 percent to 20 percent of patients, tumors shrink to less than half their original size, and for many of these patients the tumors disappear and don't grow back. According to the American Cancer Society, "IL-2 is the only therapy that appears to result in long-lasting responses." In addition to skipping over these benefits of IL-2, Ken's doctor also glossed over the downside of Sutent, the drug he wanted Ken to take. Sutent can cause long-term fatigue, and Ken feared this more than almost anything else, because his wife had leukemia and he needed to stay alert to help care for her.

In the end, Ken decided to go with IL-2, which stopped his cancer from spreading for about a year and didn't cause the long-term fatigue he so wanted to avoid. I spoke to him about two years after he'd finished taking IL-2, and although the cancer hadn't disappeared, he was feeling well and active—and he was grateful he'd had the energy to care for his wife, who eventually succumbed to her cancer. Although it didn't cure his cancer, Ken knows IL-2 was the right choice for him, and he's glad he found it. "The doctor I saw was one of the leading renal oncologists in the world," he told me. "If I hadn't done my Internet research, I wouldn't have known about IL-2."

FAY SUTTON: Like Ken Youner, Fay Sutton learned of a treatment for her cancer not from her doctor but from the Internet. In 2004, Mrs. Sutton was diagnosed with squamous cell carcinoma, a type of skin cancer. A dermatologist suggested surgery, the standard treatment for invasive squamous cell carcinoma. But Mrs. Sutton's daughter, Dorothy, was concerned that her frail, eighty-nine-year-old mother might not survive surgery, so she sought a second opinion. The second dermatologist suggested a series of radiation treatments, but added that this approach would also be hard for Mrs. Sutton, given her age.

Dorothy Sutton sought help from Jan Guthrie, whose business, The Health Resource, does research for people with health problems. Guthrie set out to see if there were any other treatments besides surgery or radiation that would help Fay Sutton. After poking around online, she found articles by two sets of doctors, one in Germany and the other in the United States, reporting success in treating squamous cell carcinoma with a topical cream called imiquimod. Dorothy took her mother to the American doctor who wrote the article, and after three months of treatment with the cream, a biopsy showed that there were no signs of cancer cells. The last time I spoke with Dorothy, her mother was ninety-three years old and cancer-free. While imiquimod isn't the first-choice treatment for most people with invasive squamous cell cancer—surgery is—it was the right treatment for Mrs. Sutton, allowing her to avoid surgery and radiation.

WHAT THE STUDIES SAY

Not surprisingly, each year studies show that more and more people are going online to obtain health information, to the point where nearly everyone with an Internet connection is now searching for answers to their health questions, just as they go online to do their banking or their Christmas shopping. And we patients aren't just searching for answers online; we're finding them. According to a 2009 report by the Pew Internet & American Life Project, 60 percent of Internet users said the information they found online affected a decision about how to treat an illness or a condition, 53 percent said online information had led them to ask a doctor new questions or to get a second opinion, and 38 percent said what they learned online changed the way they cope with a chronic condition or manage pain.

While patients find the Internet extremely useful, the flip side is many doctors find it to be a major annoyance. A 2003 survey of more than 1,000 physicians showed that 38 percent believed that when a patient brings in information from the Internet, it makes the visit less time-efficient. In focus groups, doctors have used words like "hard time," "headache," "nightmare," "annoying," "irritating," and "frustrating" to describe their experiences with Internet-educated patients. Getting information online, the doctors said, made patients feel "anxious," "worried," "nervous," and "panicked," and sometimes "overwhelmed" and "sicker." This report is titled "Are Physicians Ready for Patients with Internet-Based Health Information?," and the answer appears to be "No." The researchers found many physicians felt that when patients did "self-misdiagnosis" on the Internet they (the doctors) then had to do "substantial work" to debunk "incorrect information." Furthermore, these doctors felt they had to justify themselves when their professional diagnosis differed from what patients found online. "In having their expertise challenged, some physicians felt they were at risk of 'losing face' and/or being 'put on the spot,' " the authors of the study observed.

Several doctors have expressed themselves quite publicly about their distaste for Internet-educated patients. Writing in *The Journal of the American Medical Association,* one doctor lamented, "Our patients are turning to electronic resources as their primary source of medical information [where] irrelevant and inaccurate information . . . leads to all kinds of confusing philosophies. Medicine is no place for confusing philosophies." Another doctor, writing in the *Archives of Surgery,* complained, "A little knowledge truly is a bad thing." This surgeon bemoaned patients who go on the Internet before coming to see him, as "this can contribute to mistrust and, ultimately, may compromise the appropriate provision of health care." Like the physicians in the survey, this surgeon—a young guy, by the way, not some pre-Internet curmudgeon—complained about the "lengthy reeducation" doctors must do when patients have been miseducated online. Another physician employed a particularly simple solution for patients coming in with Internet printouts: "Most [patients] know it's annoying to me when they do it, so they don't."

I recently went on Twitter and asked my legions of doctor followers why they thought the Internet made doctors so grouchy. A doctor for whom I have a good deal of respect tweeted back, "The role of the expert is to know what to ignore. Printouts often irrelevant. Distract from real issue." I think I understand what she means: patients bring in all sorts of stuff from the Internet that has nothing to do with their illness, and the expert—the doctor—knows on her own what's important. I can see where this would be true in many instances, when patients bring in extraneous information and the doctor's explaining why it's useless steals away precious minutes in the examining room. The experiences of Marian Sandmaier, Ken Youner, and Fay Sutton (and two people we met in chapter 4, Marci Smith and Trisha Torrey, who corrected their doctors' incorrect cancer diagnoses with Internet information) show that patients are gleaning invaluable health information online. The trick is recognizing relevant information and presenting it to your doctor in a way that he finds useful rather than threatening.

SOLUTIONS: HOW TO HARNESS THE HEALTH POWER
OF THE INTERNET

While doctors may not like the Internet, you're smart and you know it's full of powerful advice and solutions for your health problems. Despite all the agonizing from the folks I call Internet Eeyores about the dangers of these quack sites—and there *is* a lot of garbage on the Internet—I really don't think it's terribly difficult to separate the good health sites from the bad. First, there are some sites that are clearly reliable. Sites with ".gov" or ".edu" at the end of the address are generally trustworthy, as they're run by a government agency or a university. Established groups, like the American Heart Association or the American Cancer Society, also have trustworthy websites, and respected news sites like cnnhealth.com are well-vetted sources of information.

You'll need to use your common sense in evaluating other sites that are less well-known. One big red flag is when a website is trying to sell you a product; I'm extremely wary of these. Sometimes it's clear that a site is hawking something (the big advertisements are your first clue), but at other times it may be more subtle. That's why if you're unfamiliar with a website you should click on "About Us." This section, or something like it, will hopefully tell you who runs the site and who funds it, which is important to know. For example, some patient-advocacy sites look as if they're 100 percent about patients when they're actually funded by a drug company, and you'd learn that only by reading the fine print. I wouldn't necessarily jettison everything on that site, but I'd take what I read with a grain of salt.

The Top Five Reasons You Need to Go Beyond Google

1. You can find information being presented at medical conferences six months to a year before your doctor hears about it.

2. You can meet people with your illness and learn what they did to get better.

3. You can learn who the big researchers are for the problem you have and contact them with your questions.

4. You can find medical journal articles your doctor might never read.

5. You can learn how to read the medspeak in those articles.

GOING BEYOND GOOGLE

Two-thirds of all Internet health searchers start their online journey by typing their query into a search engine, such as Google. Google really is the perfect tool for many health questions. I'm a huge fan of Google. I use it all the time. I bet I'm one of its best customers. Just the other day, when my two-year-old had a fever and I took her temperature under her arm (since she can't reliably hold a thermometer in her mouth), I knew I was supposed to either add a degree or subtract a degree to her armpit temperature to get her true temperature, but I couldn't remember which, so there I was, holding a thermometer that read 99.6, unsure whether my daughter was okay because her temperature was really 98.6, or whether she was sick with a fever of 100.6 degrees. With Yaara on one knee and my laptop on the other, I Googled "baby armpit temperature" and voilà, there it was, a reliable site telling me to add a degree (and to check the temperature rectally, since under the arm isn't the most accurate method). It took me exactly thirty seconds to find this out (I timed myself), and since I'm a paranoid mommy I corroborated the information on two more sites just to make sure it was right, which took me another minute at the most. In about ninety seconds I had my answer, and I knew that my daughter likely did have a fever. Thank you, Dr. Google!

Google is great for finding answers to such simple questions, but for many problems a Google search simply isn't enough. For example, if Dorothy Sutton had just Googled "treatments for skin cancer" when her mother was diagnosed, she would never have found imiquimod, the cream that cured her mother's cancer. The two studies that mentioned imiquimod as a skin-cancer treatment were only in relatively obscure medical journals and would likely never have popped up on a Google search.

To find the imiquimod solution, Dorothy needed to know how to Go Beyond Google, or GBG, as I like to call it. Going Beyond Google isn't hard, and boy, is it worth it. When I teach you how to GBG, you'll find out about new medical discoveries six months to a year before your doctor hears about them. You'll find solutions to your medical problems that your doctor hasn't even heard about yet. You'll be able to catch a doctor's misdiagnosis. You'll know how to get in touch with the top experts in any given field. Once you learn how to GBG, you'll truly be able to harness the incredible health power of the Internet.

The first step in Going Beyond Google is to get an overview of the health problem you're researching so you can then zero in on that one piece of information that might be helpful to you. To do this, use a search engine like Dirline (www.dirline.nlm.nih.gov) or MedlinePlus (www.medlineplus.gov), both run by the National Library of Medicine, which give you good general information without the garbage often included in a Google search. Another good place to start is with a review article about your particular problem. Review articles give a good overview of the latest research in a particular area. You can find review articles by going to PubMed (www.pubmed.gov), which is also run by the National Library of Medicine. Go to the "Limits" tab and then under "Type of Article" check "Review." Tara Parker-Pope, of *The New York Times,* who suggested this technique to me, said she found review articles helpful when her mother was first diagnosed with cancer.

Another good way to find the latest medical research is to check out medical conferences, as researchers often announce their latest discoveries at professional conferences many months or even years before they publish these discoveries in the medical journals your doctor reads. To find a medical organization that's pertinent to your particular health problem, go to the American Medical Association's list of medical societies; the URL is long and complicated, so it's easiest just to Google "AMA National Medical Specialty Society Websites" and you'll get right there. MedlinePlus has one, too—Google "MedlinePlus all organizations." It's usually pretty clear which medical society you want: cancer researchers present their findings to groups like the American Cancer Society, heart docs speak at the annual meeting of the American College of Cardiology, etc.

Another technique for Going Beyond Google is to recognize that other people have had your disease, and many of them are whip-smart and online. For example, in chapter 2 we met Erica Gero, who says that she owes her life to a patient she met on the Association of Cancer Online Resources (www.acor.org). Patients on sites like ACOR are an invaluable source of collective wisdom. Use them.

Speaking of wise patients, when you have a medical question find a smart blogger or a smart advocacy group for your disease. As I write this, I can hear the Greek chorus of Eeyores proclaiming that you couldn't *possibly* rely on a *blogger*—a *common* person—to give you reliable information about a health issue. To that I say, "Oh, please." Of course there are idiots out there blogging, but there are also really smart folks who keep up with the latest research, often attending conferences your doctor will never go to. You're a smart person, and I have faith in your ability to separate the jerks who are just mouthing off from the people who actually know what they're talking about. Just as you do when evaluating websites, use your common sense with bloggers. For example, if a blogger is selling a product ("My homemade herbal mixture cures colon cancer! Just $19.99, plus shipping and handling!") you know you should stay away.

YOU CAN READ MEDICAL JOURNAL ARTICLES!

You'll notice that much of my advice ends up with you reading studies from medical journals. Don't be scared—it's not that hard. As an example, let's go back to Dorothy Sutton, the woman who was looking for new treatments for her mom's skin cancer. Let's say Dorothy hadn't used Jan Guthrie, the professional researcher, and wanted to read the articles on her own. Let's take a look at one of these skin cancer articles, written by Dr. Keyvan Nouri and colleagues at the University of Miami School of Medicine. Medical journal articles are long and intimidating, so here's what you should do: focus on the abstract, which is the short synopsis of the study presented at the beginning of the article. If that doesn't work, go to the end of the study and read the conclusion. In the case of Dr. Nouri's article, which appears in the *Journal of Drugs in Dermatology*, the abstract has everything we need. Take a look at this section:

> There have . . . been some case reports and case series reporting success treating squamous cell carcinoma in situ with imiquimod. We report two patients with squamous cell carcinoma in situ and one with invasive squamous cell carcinoma treated with 5% imiquimod cream. Lesions were located on shin, posterior shoulder, and nasal tip. 5% imiquimod cream was applied at night for six weeks. Side effects included erythema and crusting in one patient. Biopsies taken four weeks after treatment revealed no residual squamous cell carcinoma in situ or squamous cell carcinoma. Topical 5% imiquimod cream is becoming established as a promising treatment for squamous cell carcinoma in situ. It also seems to be an alternative treatment for some cases of squamous cell carcinoma.

Sound like Greek to you? Don't worry—you can decipher it by using something I call the Russian-Novel Approach. You know how in a Russian novel you just mentally bleep out all the long five-syllable names you can't understand? Do the same thing here. So if you don't know what "case reports," "case series," and "in situ" mean, bleep them out and you'll get "reporting success treating of squamous cell carcinoma with imiquimod." That's easy to understand—and it sounds promising, right? Here's another sentence that mentions Mrs. Sutton's disease: "Biopsies taken four weeks after treatment revealed no residual squamous cell carcinoma in situ or squamous cell carcinoma. Topical 5% imiquimod cream is becoming established as a promising treatment for squamous cell carcinoma in situ. It also seems to be an alternative treatment for some cases of squamous cell carcinoma." Do the Russian-novel thing and you get: "no residual squamous cell carcinoma. . . . Imiquimod cream is becoming established as a promising treatment for squamous cell carcinoma . . . an alternative treatment for some cases of squamous cell carcinoma." Maybe Dorothy Sutton wouldn't have understood this completely, but she would have understood the gist of it, comprehending enough to say to a doctor, "Hey, I read a study online about imiquimod for Mom's type of cancer. Might it work for her instead of surgery or radiation?"

By the way, if you want to know what some of those Russian-novel terms mean, I recommend "Deciphering Medspeak" from the Medical Library Association. Again, it's a complicated URL, so just Google "MLA Deciphering Medspeak."

EMAILING DOCTORS YOU DON'T KNOW

So let's say Dorothy Sutton had found, read, and understood Dr. Nouri's article online. She's ecstatic—this is the holy grail! Finally, a solution for her mom! Now what does she do? Dorothy could take Dr. Nouri's journal article to her doctor for discussion, but I have to tell you, I think she's going to get some serious eye rolling if she does this. As we've seen, doctors often dismiss novel approaches patients find online. (Allow me to get on my soapbox here for a moment: I'm always amazed when doctors roll their eyes, completely dismissing "stuff patients find online," as if every single thing on the Internet were garbage or quackery. Aren't they aware that real medical journals—*The New England Journal of Medicine, The Journal of the American Medical Association,* for example—put their articles online? Don't they know that the American Cancer Society and the American Heart Association have websites? Aren't they legitimate? Why is something automatically tainted if it's found online?)

Now that I'm off my soapbox, back to the Suttons. Let's say Fay Sutton's doctor had been receptive to the article about imiquimod and had read it thoroughly. There's still a good chance he might not have wanted to use imiquimod, as it was a new approach in the treatment of skin cancer and not widely accepted. Where would that have left the Suttons? In this case, Dorothy and Fay Sutton were very lucky; they live near the University of Miami, where Dr. Nouri works, so they left their doctor and just went to see Dr. Nouri. But what if the Suttons had lived in, say, Oregon? Here's a little secret your doctor won't tell you: physicians, especially those who are leaders in their field, will often read and respond to emails from people they've never heard of. Dorothy Sutton could have emailed Dr. Nouri asking his advice about imiquimod, and if he had recommended trying the cream, she could have shared that with her own doctor. In fact, she could have asked Dr. Nouri to get on the phone with her doctor to educate him about this new approach to skin cancer.

I used to think doctors would never respond to emails from patients they didn't know, but I've learned that I'm wrong. While doing research for an "Empowered Patient" column after the death of Senator Edward Kennedy, my colleague David Martin, a senior producer on CNN's medical team, spoke to two neurosurgeons who weren't the senator's doctors but had nonetheless advised him on how to treat his cancer. You're probably thinking, Yeah, sure a doctor will respond to a request from a Kennedy, but I'm not a Kennedy, and they'll probably ignore an email from me. But the two surgeons David spoke with said they often respond to emails from patients they don't know. Dr. Raymond Sawaya, chairman of the Department of Neurosurgery at the M. D. Anderson Cancer Center and Baylor College of Medicine in Houston, noted that "smart people write to the top four or five major centers in the country." What should you say in an email to an expert? Jan Guthrie, the researcher who helped the Suttons, writes these kinds of emails quite often and has some advice: "Stroke them a little and say you read their article and how much you enjoyed their study. Don't write three or four paragraphs. Just ask your question." Guthrie said that she sent a blind email to a cancer specialist when she herself was diagnosed with ovarian cancer, and she got a helpful response; she still emails this doctor with questions from time to time.

If your illness is serious and you can afford it, you can even consider making a trip to the doctor you've met online. While doing research for a woman with a rare type of liver tumor, Guthrie found a doctor who had done extensive work on her type of tumor. This doctor worked in New York, and the woman with the tumor lived in Arizona. "She went to New York once, and this specialist stayed on her team," Guthrie says. "They email each other, and the New York doctor consults with the doctor in Arizona. If you're easy to work with and not difficult, they'll stay in touch with you."

How would you find a doctor's email? Here's where Going Beyond Google comes in handy once again. In chapter 4, we talked a bit about finding a doctor's email address, but let's go into more detail here. Let's go back to Dorothy Sutton sitting on her home computer, reading Dr. Nouri's article in the *Journal of Drugs in Dermatology*. The abstract (which is free) clearly identifies Dr. Nouri as working at the University of Miami School of Medicine. But just Googling for Dr. Nouri's email wouldn't have helped. I know, because I just Googled "email Nouri Miami university" and came up with a few mentions of Dr. Nouri (plus a lot of information about the Iraqi prime minister Nouri al-Maliki) but, alas, not the doctor's email address. However, when I went to the home page for the University of Miami and put his name in its internal search engine, his email address popped right up. It took some work, and I had to GBG, but I found it!

When this university technique fails—and sometimes it does— here's another way to go beyond Google and find a doctor's email address. Go to Google Scholar and type in "email Nouri University Miami." The very first study that pops up has his email address. In this case, you don't even have to click on the study itself—the address is right there on the Google Scholar results page. If you ever do have to click on a study to find a doctor's email, just do a search for the word "correspondence" and the email address should be there.

I use these tricks all the time to find doctors' email addresses, but every so often they fail and I have to use a resource that you can't use: the CNN librarians. These crackerjack researchers are a godsend. In nearly twenty years of asking them for the most obscure pieces of information, the librarians never come up short, so I asked one of them, Krista Kordt, for advice on how laypeople can find a doctor's email address. She had a great idea. If the doctor you're looking for works for a university that doesn't list his email, go to the public-relations section of the university's website (it might be called "Media Relations" or "Newsroom"). Find addresses for its PR people and see if they follow a certain format, such as *firstname.lastname@university.edu*. Using the doctor's name, you can follow the same format.

DON'T BECOME A CYBERCHONDRIAC

Compared with Edwin Murphy, the patient who had to impersonate a doctor in order to get the health information he needed, we're
all blessed many times over. With the right skills, we can access
practically any medical information we want anytime we want.
With such blessings, however, comes a curse: the curse of cyberchondria. With so much information available, you might start to
convince yourself that you have a deadly disease when you really
just have some minor ailment. You know what I mean: you have a
headache, start Googling around, and within minutes become convinced you've got a brain tumor. It's similar to a well-known disorder that predates the Internet called medical student syndrome,
where doctors in training become convinced they have every disease they read about in their textbooks. Every mole on their body
is skin cancer. A nosebleed is surely a sign of a tumor. Headache?
Must be skyrocketing blood pressure. On the Internet, it's pretty
easy to become that scared medical student.

Thankfully, you can learn to avoid cyberchondria. Dr. Arthur
Barsky, a professor of psychiatry at Harvard Medical School who
has treated cyberchondriacal patients, has some advice. First, be
very clear about what you're trying to learn on the Internet—don't
go on a fishing expedition. "Plan in advance what you want to find
out, what the question is you're trying to answer, and how much
time you're willing to spend on it," Dr. Barsky advises. "If you find
yourself exceeding those limits, you should ratchet it down."

And here's some advice from Dr. Vicki Rackner, a patient advocate who herself suffered from medical student syndrome when
she was in school. "I was studying for an exam on the pancreas, and
I became convinced that I had a rare type of pancreatic tumor,"
Rackner recalls. "I thought, I don't need to study because I'm going
to die." What snapped her out of it? A good night's sleep and an
honest discussion with herself. "When you're off on a medical

wild-goose chase, you disconnect yourself from your intuition. Ask yourself, do you really have this disease? The answer will almost always be 'No.' "

The Case of the Tingling Hands

Take a minute and Google "tingling hands." Within seconds you'll find that a tingling sensation in your hands could mean you have AIDS, anxiety, arsenic poisoning, leprosy, or something called Besnier-Boeck-Schaumann disease.

Here's why you shouldn't panic. "Understand that it is common to have 'all the symptoms' of something and not have it," says Dr. Robert Lamberts, a family physician in Augusta, Georgia, and a medical blogger. In the case of the tingling hands, it's far more likely you have anxiety than arsenic poisoning. Hypothyroidism is another example. "The symptoms are weight gain and fatigue. Throw in constipation and dry skin and you are down to about one-third of the U.S. population," says Dr. Lamberts. Of course, only a small percentage of people with weight gain, fatigue, constipation, and dry skin actually have hypothyroidism.

NOW FOR THE HARD PART

So now you know how to harness the full power of the Internet. You search out medical journal articles like a pro, and you can actually understand them. You've gained the confidence to email doctors you don't know and ask your medical questions. You even know how to make sure you don't slip into cyberchondria.

But you still haven't done the hard part: getting your doctor to pay attention to what you've found online. As we've seen, you may be proud as punch at the medical jewels you've found online, but there's an excellent chance your doctor will just roll his eyes at you.

There are several ways of handling this situation. If your doctor is truly dismissive of the information you've learned, you can leave him and find another doctor. But if you want to stick with your physician (or if he's your only option), there are ways to work around a doctor's dismissive attitude. First, don't present Internet information as a challenge or a demand. "Internet junkies who come to their appointment armed with stacks of Internet searches and loaded for bear are unlikely to have a rewarding visit," Dr. John Castaldo, chief of the Division of Neurology at Lehigh Valley Hospital in Pennsylvania, wrote in the journal *Neurology Today*. Instead of coming "loaded for bear," ask your doctor for his expertise in helping you to interpret what you've found on the Internet. "Don't say, 'Well, I looked it up on the Internet, and I think it is X.' Instead say: 'Doctor, what do you think about X? I heard about it and it sounds like I have some of the symptoms,' " Dr. Lamberts advises.

Be sure to vet websites before showing them to your doctor. If a website is selling a product, or is the only site on the Internet making a certain claim ("Grapefruit juice opens blocked arteries!"), don't waste a doctor's time with it. When you find websites you do like and trust, don't just fork the printouts over to your doctor. If you do, you're effectively saying, "Here, go through these," when the doctor has a waiting room full of patients to see. Instead, make bullet points of the information you found, or find one website that concisely explains what you want to convey to your doctor and print out just that one item. "Boil down your links" is how Dr. Charles Smith, a family practitioner in Arkansas and the founder of the website edocamerica.com, puts it. He had a great idea: ask your doctor for his email address and explain that it might be quicker and easier if you could send your bullet points in a follow-up email, along with links to the websites you've read. "A lot of this is more easily done in email," he told me. "I do this with a lot of my patients, and I'll look at it when I have five or ten minutes. It's very quick for me to do after the office has shut down."

CONCLUSION

While many doctors still take a dismissive attitude toward health information on the Internet, I think it's going to become more and more uncool for docs to diss online information. One young physician, Dr. Manjula Gunawardane, actually wrote admiringly of the Internet: "Patients are bypassing [an] outdated system and finding novel ways to utilize the Web to manage their illnesses, bolster their medical knowledge, and provide support to others." And check out the title of this paper by Dr. Corey Siegel at Dartmouth Medical School: "Embracing the Internet for Progress in Shared Decision-Making." How refreshing! Hedy Wald, who teaches medical students at Brown University, has urged doctors to get with the program. "Welcome to the world of Web savvy patients—they're already navigating cyberspace with ease and you just might want to get on board," she and her colleagues wrote in a medical journal. "The clothing retailer's motto 'An educated consumer is our best customer' may hold true for the field of medicine as well. Collaborative teamwork between physician and patient might just lead to a genuine partnership, improving the quality of health care and engendering a more trusting physician-patient relationship. Might be worth a try." In an article in *Neurology Today,* Dr. Castaldo, the neurologist and a co-author of the book *The Man with the Iron Tattoo,* advised his colleagues: "Accept the fact that the Internet is here to stay. . . . Take their health care Internet searches seriously and don't deride or denigrate their efforts. Informed patients are better patients." Dr. Smith, the family doctor in Arkansas, says he's *grateful* when patients do Internet research, especially when the patient has an unusual disease that he might not have seen very often in his practice. "I have a million things to worry about, and he has one," Dr. Smith told me. "He's intelligent and on the Internet, and he can put hundreds of hours into research that a physician just wouldn't have."

After more than a decade of hearing doctors whine about the Internet, it's nothing short of miraculous that they're beginning to recognize the power the Internet holds for improving our health. I think Dr. Castaldo put it best when he wrote to his colleagues, "You will find your patients sometimes will surprise you with what they know and can in fact teach you a thing or two. This is okay. The doctor-patient relationship includes the teacher learning from the student. Take joy in that."

Remember that I told you how I went on Twitter and asked doctors why they were so irked by patients who come into the office with Internet printouts? Well, I was surprised to receive tweets from several physicians saying this didn't bother them at all, that they actually liked it when patients brought in information they'd found online. I think you're still going to find doctors who bristle at the sight of a patient with printouts, but my guess is, with more doctors coming around to Dr. Castaldo's way of thinking, this holiday season the American Medical Association won't be warning patients to stay away from the Internet.

Final Checklist: How to Become an Internet MD (Medical Detective)

1. **Separate the good health sites from the bad.** There's a lot of garbage on the Internet, and you need to learn how to weed it out. You can generally trust sites that end in ".gov" or ".edu" and sites that belong to well-established groups such as the American Heart Association or the American Cancer Society. For other sites, click on "About Us" to find out who runs it. One way to avoid Internet misinformation is to use search engines that filter out the garbage, such as Dirline (www.dirline.nlm.nih.gov) and MedlinePlus (www.medlineplus.gov), both of which are run by the National Library of Medicine. Be wary of sites that are trying to sell you a product.

2. **Find patients like yourself.** If you've just been diagnosed with a disease, you can learn a great deal from people who have had your disease for years. Search out sites where smart patients talk to one another, and look for intelligent bloggers who have your disease. Many are happy to answer your questions, and you can find out what they did to get better.

3. **Go Beyond Google.** Google is good for quick, easy questions, but for anything more complex learn how to dig deeper for your answers. To get the latest, cutting-edge medical information, you need to learn how to go beyond Google to find information that your doctor may not learn about for months!

4. **Go directly to the original medical research.** Google Scholar (www.google.com/scholar) and PubMed (www.pubmed .gov) will get you right to the medical journal articles you need to read. Invest thirty minutes in taking the PubMed tutorial and read review articles to get an overview of the latest medical research on your disease.

5. **To read a medical journal article, utilize the Russian-Novel Approach.** When you're reading an article in a medical journal, read the abstract and, if you need to, the conclusion. If you don't understand a word, just bleep it out, as we all do with the five-syllable names in Russian novels. Even if you understand only the gist of what you're reading in an article, I bet it'll be enough to allow you to ask your doctor questions. If you do want to know what a medical term means, read "Deciphering Medspeak" from the Medical Library Association.

6. **Read information being presented at medical conferences.** Researchers generally present their work at conferences six months to a year before they publish it in a journal. Go to the website for the medical society that's related to your disease and look up the abstracts being presented at its annual conference.

7. **Email physicians who are leaders in their field to get their advice.** Once you start reading journal articles and conference abstracts, you'll begin to see who the leaders in the field are. You don't have to be that doctor's patient to send him an email. Just send it; many doctors tell me they respond to emails from patients they don't know.

8. **Learn how to find a doctor's email address.** If the doctor you want to email works at a university, go to the school's website and do a search for his name. If it's not there, or if the doctor doesn't work for a university, look up the name on Google Scholar or PubMed. The author's email address is almost always published in the study.

9. **Don't become a cyberchondriac.** Let's say you have a headache. If Googling around convinces you that it's due to a brain tumor, you've slipped into cyberchondria. Set time limits when you do health research on the Internet, and stay focused. Don't go off on a medical wild-goose chase—be very clear with yourself about what you're trying to figure out.

10. **Don't throw a stack of Internet printouts at your doctor.** Boil down the information you've learned into bullet points and discuss those with your doctor. Choose your words carefully. Don't say, "Well, I looked it up on the Internet and I think it's X." Instead, say, "Doctor, what do you think about X? I have heard about it, and I wonder if that's what I have."

CHAPTER SIX

You vs. the Insurance Industry

Patsy Bates was cutting a client's hair at a salon in Southern California when an insurance salesman walked in, all smiles, touting his newest policies. Patsy told him to come on in; she had health insurance but was interested in hearing if he might have something better for her.

After listening to the sales pitch, Patsy was impressed. This new policy seemed to cover much more than the policy she had, and it was less expensive to boot. The salesman whipped out an application and asked Patsy a few questions and, since she was cutting hair, filled in the answers for her. Patsy signed the form and soon received a packet in the mail welcoming her to the Health Net insurance family.

Later, Patsy would say signing on that dotted line was the biggest mistake of her life. A few months after joining Health Net, Patsy was diagnosed with breast cancer, and the company dropped her policy right in the middle of the chemotherapy treatments. Her doctors refused to continue seeing her, and Patsy was left with no chemotherapy and $100,000 in bills. "I shed a lot of tears, and I just prayed a lot," she told me when I visited her at her hair salon in Gardena, California. "I said, 'Lord, what do I do?'" She signed up for Medicaid, and had to go without her chemo until the application went through.

When Patsy asked a customer-service representative at Health

Net why her policy was canceled, she was told that she hadn't been truthful on her application. If you lie about something important on an insurance application, it really is legitimate for the company to drop you. For example, if you say you don't have cancer when you really were diagnosed with cancer six months ago, you can kiss that insurance policy goodbye the day you go in for treatment. Fair or not, insurance companies can legally cancel your policy if they figure out that you're seeking care for a condition you knew you had but said you didn't.

In Patsy's case, though, Health Net had some pretty flimsy reasons for canceling her policy. She was accused of shaving a few pounds off her weight on the application, and she neglected to mention she'd had heart-valve problems a decade earlier, and that she'd recently gone to the emergency room for chest pain. Patsy explained to Health Net that weight, heart-valve problems, and chest pain have nothing to do with breast cancer. Second, she explained she'd answered the salesman's questions honestly. He'd asked if she had any major illnesses, and she didn't. Her heart-valve problems had gone away, and the doctors in the emergency room told her the chest pain was nothing to worry about and sent her home. As for her weight, Patsy explained that she'd given the salesman her best guess.

In a landmark case, Patsy Bates sued Health Net and won. The judge in the case, Sam Cianchetti, raked Health Net over the coals for canceling her policy in the middle of her chemotherapy on such a ridiculous pretext. "It's hard to imagine a situation more trying than the one Bates had to endure," Cianchetti wrote. "Health Net's conduct was reprehensible." Patsy was awarded $9 million.

THE MURRAY FAMILY: CAUGHT IN A SCAM

I often hear from people who are having problems with their health insurance, and I've had some of my own, so I can understand where they're coming from. First, it's really hard to figure out which kind of insurance to get in the first place, whether you're selecting from a list of options provided by your employer or buying insurance on your own. Second, when you're shopping for insurance on your own, there are all sorts of scammers out there waiting to take advantage of you. Third, as we can see from Patsy Bates's experience, even when you have insurance, you're not safe, because the company can drop you or refuse to pay the bills and you're left on your own, David fighting Goliath.

Let me tell you about the scams first. For my "Empowered Patient" column, we interviewed Hope Murray, a California woman who saw an advertisement on the Internet for a medical discount card. She initially thought her prayers had been answered. Hope's daughter, Meredith, desperately needed to see a doctor after suffering a brain injury in a car accident, but she was in graduate school and didn't have insurance. When Meredith applied for insurance, no company would take her because of her preexisting condition. The card advertised $30 doctor visits and $50 visits to specialists, and Hope Murray immediately signed up. "It was pretty phenomenal," she said. "They promised me everything was included," including doctor visits, vision, dental, and hospital stays. "They even mentioned the Mayo Clinic."

Hope paid $314 up front for her daughter's card and then $179 each following month. But when Meredith tried to actually use the card, things didn't go so well. She called a doctor listed on the card's website, but that doctor had never even heard of the discount card. Meredith called another doctor listed on the card's website, and then another and another. None of them had heard of the card, and none of them offered any kind of discount. At CNN, my colleagues and I were immediately suspicious. CNN's senior medical producer Jennifer Bixler called several physicians the site listed as accepting discounts, and they'd also never heard of the card. The "discount card" company had made it all up.

"I have never been more angry, more furious, about anything in my life," Hope told me. "It is a bogus scam that hurts people. It should be a crime for people to do that." She canceled the card three months after signing up. By that time, she'd spent more than $850 on a card that had given her absolutely nothing. Like most people, Hope never sued the card company; it would have cost her way more than $850 to take the case to court. Hope says she learned her lesson. Now that her daughter has graduated from school, she's on her way to a job that offers insurance—real insurance—so that she can take care of her health problems.

WHAT THE STUDIES SAY: CHOOSING INSURANCE WISELY

After talking with Hope Murray, I called Jim Quiggle, a spokesman for the Coalition Against Insurance Fraud. "Have you ever heard of these things?" I asked him. Boy, had he ever. "Medical discount cards are spreading like kudzu," Quiggle told me. "There's a tremendous amount of fraud and deception in these plans." He told me that the Federal Trade Commission and at least eight states have taken action against more than two dozen so-called medical discount cards for offering services that don't exist.

Discount cards aren't the only scam out there. There are also companies trying to sell fake health insurance that "isn't worth the paper it's written on," Quiggle says. Between 2000 and 2002, the Government Accountability Office found that at least 144 companies had been identified as selling fake coverage to more than 200,000 policyholders—leaving at least $252 million in unpaid medical claims.

In this chapter I'll teach you how to avoid the kind of scam that soaked the Murrays. I'll also show you how to challenge your insurance company when it tries to cheat you, which happened to Patsy Bates. Finally, I'll walk you through the steps involved in buying health-care insurance.

SOLUTIONS, PART 1: HOW TO AVOID INSURANCE SCAMS

When you're shopping for health insurance, you need to keep your guard up for three different potentially problematic situations. First, all the experts I talked to recommend avoiding discount cards, like the one Hope Murray purchased, altogether. They say many are total rip-offs, that even if the card is legit and offers true discounts, the discounts aren't that great, and—most important— the card isn't insurance. It's not going to foot the bill—or even a substantial part of it—if disaster strikes.

The National Association of Insurance Commissioners recommends a high degree of vigilance when buying a discount card. First of all, it's a big red flag if a discount card is advertised in an Internet pop-up ad or fax blast. Also, be wary of terms like "guaranteed coverage." When you're looking into a card, ask for a list of providers and then call those providers to make sure they really do take the card. If the card company won't give you a list of providers, don't buy the card. Finally, nail down the numbers. If a card promises you a 30 percent discount off doctors' visits, this means absolutely nothing—you need to ask 30 percent off what? That's why you need to call the doctor's office directly to get the final price.

The second kind of scam to look out for is fake insurance policies from fly-by-night companies that will disappear with your premiums as soon as you've paid them. As Steve Luptak, the executive director of a group called Healthcare Advocacy, puts it, "Will the company be in business when you need it or is it 'Shifting Sands Mutual'?" To find out if an insurance company is legit, contact your state insurance commissioner to see if it's licensed in the state. To find your state insurance office, Google "NAIC state map" to see a list of state insurance offices from the National Association of Insurance Commissioners. Also, check to see if your policy has been accredited by the National Committee for Quality Assurance (ncqa.org), a group that takes a rigorous look at policies to make sure they meet certain standards.

Once you know a prospective insurance company is legit, find out what others think about it. The National Committee for Quality Assurance has a state-by-state health-plan report card and, together with *U.S. News & World Report,* ranks the nation's best plans. Consumer Reports surveys tens of thousands of consumers to find out what they think of their health plans. (Google "Consumer Reports best health insurance.") You should also pay another visit to the National Association of Insurance Commissioners website for a state-by-state listing of consumer complaints against insurance companies. (To get there, Google "NAIC Consumer Information Service.") To learn more about what customers think about a certain policy, go to the website for J. D. Power and Associates and check out its national satisfaction survey. (The website is www .jdpower.com, and you click on the insurance tab at the top.) Finally, it's worth finding out whether the insurance company you're considering will have the financial strength to pay your claims if you get sick. Go to ehealthinsurance.com, look up your policy, and next to it there will be a financial rating from a company called A. M. Best.

The third situation you want to be very suspicious about is short-term insurance. Many people are tempted to buy it. Here's how it often happens: You graduate from college without a job, but since you're sure you're going to get one soon you don't want to spend the money on a regular health-insurance policy. You look around on the Internet and find a six-month policy for a lot less. You buy it, but you're still unemployed after six months, or the only job you can find doesn't offer insurance, so you renew for another six months. Sounds like a good plan, right? Here's the catch: you're not actually renewing your policy every six months; technically, you're buying a whole new policy. The reason this is important is that when you buy a new plan the insurance company is free to discriminate against you for preexisting conditions. This can be disastrous, and here's an example: Let's say on January 1 you buy a six-month policy and on February 1 you're diagnosed with asthma. The insurance will pay for you to have your asthma treated for the next five months, but come July 1, technically what you have is a whole new policy and the insurance company will treat your asthma as a preexisting condition and may refuse to pay for it. Karen Tumulty, a *Time* magazine writer, wrote about her brother's heartbreaking experience with short-term insurance, and it's worth going online to read the full story. (Google "The Health-Care Crisis Hits Home.") In a nutshell, Pat Tumulty faithfully paid premiums to a health-insurance company for six years, buying one six-month policy after another and hoping that soon he'd find a job with insurance. But he never did, and when he was diagnosed with kidney failure, the company refused to pay for his care, because as soon as the six-month policy was up he was considered a new customer with a preexisting condition. If it had been a long-term policy, the company wouldn't have been able to do that. Karen, a well-known medical journalist who had hosted a presidential candidates' forum on health care, complained to the state of Texas, where her brother lives, and the insurance company agreed to pay his claims for the previous year. For her brother's future care, Karen managed to find a program for low-income patients run by the county.

All the experts I've spoken with say you should avoid short-term insurance policies like the plague. "It's never, never, never a good idea," says Nancy Metcalf, the senior program editor at *Consumer Reports.* So what do you do if you don't have a job with insurance but think you're going to find one any minute? Metcalf says you can purchase regular, long-term insurance and pay by the month. When you find work that gives you insurance, just stop paying the monthly premiums on the insurance you bought on your own.

SOLUTIONS, PART 2: HOW TO PURCHASE THE POLICY THAT IS BEST FOR YOU

Now that you know how to avoid the bad policies, here's how to select the best policy from the good ones out there. Whether you're choosing from options presented by your employer or buying a policy on your own, there are certain principles that apply to being a smart shopper. Your first step when purchasing insurance is to decide whether you want an HMO or a PPO. Generally speaking, HMOs (health-maintenance organizations) are less expensive but offer fewer choices of doctors, forcing you to stay within their provider network. PPOs (preferred-provider organizations) cost more but allow you to visit a doctor outside their network for a price. Either way, make sure you can live with the choice of doctors who are in network or, in the case of the PPO, make sure you can afford to go out of network.

Once you've settled on a relatively small number of prospective policies, ask yourself these four questions about each plan:

1. How much will I pay in premiums for this plan? Think of premiums as the price tag for purchasing the plan. Everyone pays premiums, usually once a month, whether you get sick or not.

2. What will my deductible be? For most policies, at the beginning of the year the insurance company won't pay a cent for your medical care. You have to pay for everything up to a certain point. That point is called the deductible. Let's say your deductible is $1,000. This means you'll have to pay the first $1,000 of your medical costs; after that, the insurance will kick in and start paying its share. The size of the deductible varies with each plan.

3. Once I've met my deductible, what portion of the bills will I be responsible for? Once you've met your deductible, chances are

your insurance still won't pay 100 percent of your medical bills; you'll have to pay out of your own pocket for a portion of every charge. Find out what that portion is: Will you have to pay 20 percent of the charges? Ten percent? Some people (the lucky ones) don't pay a percentage and, instead, pay a flat fee—say, $20 for a visit to a doctor.

4. What will be my out-of-pocket maximum? Medical charges are so ridiculously high that at some point you won't be able to afford your 20 percent share of the bill. For example, if you become very ill it's not hard to rack up $100,000 in hospital bills. If you have a 20 percent co-pay, you'd be expected to pay $20,000 out of your own pocket. Not many people have that kind of cash sitting around, which is why policies generally place a limit on how much you're required to shell out, and after that limit, the insurance company will pay 100 percent for everything. The dollar amount of the total payment you will have to make—often called the out-of-pocket maximum or cap—depends on the policy you buy.

Once you've answered these four questions, ponder this general rule of thumb: *the higher the premiums the lower the deductible* and the lower the out-of-pocket cap, and *the lower the premiums the higher the deductible* and the higher the out-of-pocket cap. In other words, if you pay a lot up front (higher premiums), you'll likely have to dish out less money when you get sick. Conversely, if you pay less up front (lower premiums), you'll have to dish out more money when you get sick. Not surprisingly, then, the policy you choose depends on how often you get sick. For example, if you go to the doctor once a year, you probably want a policy with the lowest premiums you can find and you don't care what size the deductible is because you're never going to get close to meeting it anyway. On the other hand, if you and your family go to the doctor frequently, a high deductible could really bite you in the butt, because it means you'll need to spend a lot of money before the insurance kicks in. So in this case you might want to pay more in premiums in order to have a lower deductible (of course, there's no real way of predicting how sick you'll be in the furure).

As you can see, how sick you get plays a big role in choosing insurance. But there's one more factor at play: how nervous a person you are. I know a perfectly healthy single person at CNN who every year chooses the company's fanciest insurance plan, with the highest premiums. When I asked her why, she said she did this because she was nervous that she might get cancer or be hit by a bus or something and she didn't want to have to meet a high deductible before the insurance started to pay; she also wanted a low out-of-pocket max in case of these unforeseen disasters. While it didn't make much sense to me, she was a nervous sort of gal and was willing to pay a high premium (no pun intended) for insurance that would be more generous should she become ill.

When you make your final choice, there's one last thing to check out in the fine print: limits and exclusions. Nancy Davenport-Ennis, a co-founder of the Patient Advocate Foundation, says that some policies have pretty severe limits, such as only twelve mental-health appointments per year, or only $30,000 to treat cancer, which won't get you very far.

I don't have to tell you that choosing an insurance policy is mind-boggling. If you get insurance through your employer, I hope that your employer, like mine, does a good job of laying out all the options and helping you decide which is best for you and your family.

How to Get Help When You're Battling
Your Insurance Company

There's no question that it's a David vs. Goliath situation when your health-insurance company refuses to pay up. You can tackle the problem by yourself—many people have done so successfully—but you can also get help. Here are some sources:

1. Other patients: Others before you have argued their cases. Browse the Web for a patients' group whose members have your disease, and you can use your knowledge of what worked for them to get a denial appealed.
2. Your company's benefits office: If you get insurance through your employer, ask the benefits folks for help in reversing a denial.
3. Your doctor: There's a good chance she's had other patients with the same problem. She may be able to resubmit the claim and get it paid for.
4. The hospital's business office: It's in the hospital's interest to get paid, and it has the expertise to try to make this happen.
5. The Patient Advocate Foundation: The organization says that it gets denials reversed 94 percent of the time, and there's no charge.

SOLUTIONS, PART 3: HOW TO ARGUE
WITH YOUR INSURANCE COMPANY

Even if you follow all my advice and find the best insurance out there, you could still end up in the position Todd Robinson found himself in when his son, Bailey, was diagnosed with adrenoleukodystrophy, a rare genetic disorder that affects the brain. (It was portrayed in the movie *Lorenzo's Oil*.) Bailey died at the age of seven, but during the years of his treatment the insurance company refused to pay $200,000 in legitimate medical bills. "I don't make a lot of money," says Todd, who's a paramedic. "There's no way I could pay $200,000 out of my pocket." The Robinsons' situation isn't unusual; according to a survey by PNC Financial Services Group, one out of every four Americans has had a legitimate claim denied by an insurance company.

Just as the three most important factors in real estate are location, location, location, the three most important factors in reversing insurance denials are appeal, appeal, appeal. I know you feel as if you're in a David vs. Goliath situation when you go up against an insurance company, but appealing really does work. Todd Robinson appealed his denials, and he won back nearly every cent. You will, however, need a few slingshots in your back pocket when you fight Goliath. First, if you get your insurance through work, ask your benefits office for help. It's one thing when little ol' you asks for something, but it's quite another when the person on the other end of the phone holds the power to influence purchasing decisions for a large group. Here's an example: when my oldest daughter was a toddler, she had surgery to put tubes in her ears. The insurance company, however, claimed that a tube had been placed in only one ear and paid the surgeon only half of her fee. I politely invited the person on the other end of the phone to come on in with an otoscope and look inside my daughter's ears, because both had tubes. He declined. I argued. This went on for a year, and the bill was sent to a collection agency. Finally, I got smart and asked CNN's benefits office to make a call on my behalf, and voilà, within a few days, the surgeon got the other half of her fee.

You can also ask your doctor to fight on your behalf. A letter from her or a tweak in paperwork can make a world of difference. For example, Bailey Robinson, Todd's son, took one drug for two purposes: for chemotherapy and as treatment for anemia. The insurance wouldn't pay for the drug when it was listed as part of Bailey's chemo, so Todd asked the doctor to resubmit the claim as an anemia treatment. It worked—the insurance company paid up. In this same vein, if you have hospital charges the insurance company won't pay, you can ask the hospital's business office to give you a hand.

Last, you can get help from groups that specialize in fighting insurance companies. The Patient Advocate Foundation helped the Robinsons. "You may go through three or four levels of appeals before you get a favorable resolution," Davenport-Ennis says. (You can find her group at www.patientadvocate.org.) Also, look for advocacy groups for your specific disease, as they are there to give assistance.

In the end, the Robinsons got the insurance company's denials reversed when they wrote a threatening letter and cc'd a lawyer. "When they saw the 'Esquire' behind the names, that seemed to seal the deal," Todd told me.

Final Checklist: You and Your Health Insurance

1. **Be extremely wary of health-care discount cards.** The experts I talked to said they're a waste of money, since they're often complete scams and even the legitimate cards aren't true insurance and rarely offer much of a discount. If you still want to get one, call the doctors on the list to see if they really accept the card.

2. **Make sure an insurance company is legitimate before you purchase a policy.** Avoid fly-by-night fake insurance companies that sell bogus policies. The websites of the National Association of Insurance Commissioners and the National Committee for Quality Assurance can help you weed out scammers.

3. **Be wary of short-term insurance policies.** You might think you're going to get a job with benefits any day now, so you decide to buy a six-month insurance policy to tide you over. Experts say that's a big mistake, because each time a policy ends, the company gets to discriminate against you because of preexisting conditions. Instead, buy a long-term policy and just stop paying the monthly premiums when you don't need it anymore.

4. **When shopping for insurance, decide whether you want an HMO or a PPO.** Health-maintenance organizations generally cost less, but they also offer less flexibility when it comes to choosing a doctor. Preferred-provider organizations cost more but give you more options. Look at each policy and find out what the premiums and the deductibles will be and what percentage of costs you're expected to pay. Also, find out what the out-of-pocket max would be.

5. **Get a report card on insurance companies.** When you're out shopping for insurance and you've narrowed your options down to a few policies, find out what other people have to say about them. The National Committee for Quality Assurance has a state-by-state health-plan report card, and the National Association of Insurance Commissioners provides a state-by-state listing of consumer complaints. J. D. Power and Associates, as well as *Consumer Reports,* can give you the opinions of actual customers.

6. **When a claim is denied, appeal, appeal, appeal.** If your insurance company refuses to pay a bill it really should pay, appeal that decision. You may need to appeal multiple times before you're finally successful.

7. **When your insurance company gives you a hard time, ask for help.** When your insurance company refuses to pay legitimate claims, ask your company's benefits office for help. You can also ask your doctor or an advocacy group to step in on your behalf.

CHAPTER SEVEN

How to Get Good Drugs Cheap

Poor Bernadine. I'll never forget her. She contacted me when she saw a segment I do on CNN called "Empower Me Friday," where my colleagues and I solve viewers' health-care struggles. Bernadine sent me an email with a doozy of a problem to fix. An unemployed sixty-year-old, Bernadine was traveling from city to city in search of work and paying nearly $500 per month for prescription drugs to treat herpes, high blood pressure, and acid reflux. "I've had to stop taking one of my medicines, and I take the other two every other day or when I think I need it," Bernadine wrote to us.

To help Bernadine, I put John Bonifield, CNN's medical producer, on the case. He's one of the best diggers in the business, and I instructed him in how to go about finding Bernadine drugs that were cheaper but would still help her medical conditions. I crossed my fingers that he could find a solution. Bernadine's health depended on it.

LEE—A SIMPLE SOLUTION TO AN EXPENSIVE PROBLEM

I have some great news for you about prescription-drug prices: often it's quite easy to get your bill down. Bernadine's problem was a bit complex, as she was taking so many different drugs, so first let me tell you what I did for my friend Lee, who was a few months' pregnant when her obstetrician prescribed a prenatal vitamin called

Gesticare DHA. She went to the pharmacy and boy, did she have sticker shock: Gesticare cost $40 a month, and that was with her prescription-drug insurance. This might not sound like much, but Lee had to take these vitamins all through pregnancy and nursing, which adds up to a total price tag of at least $720.

Did she really need to pay that much? The answer is no. I made some phone calls for Lee, and I found out that she could be paying ten times less. That's right—she should have been paying $4 a month instead of $40. All she had to do was ask her doctor to switch her from Gesticare, which is a brand name, to a generic prenatal vitamin. The lesson learned here is that if you get sticker shock when you go to the pharmacy, you can call your doctor and ask if there's a less expensive drug that will work for you. Or, better yet, to avoid making that phone call, ask the right questions while you're in the doctor's office. On page 185 of the appendix, I give you a sample conversation between a doctor and a price-savvy empowered patient.

WHAT THE STUDIES SAY: WHOPPING PRESCRIPTION-DRUG PRICES

More than $100 a month for a blood-pressure medication? Nearly $200 a month to take a nightly sleeping pill? A whopping $269 a month for an antidepressant? No wonder so many Americans go bankrupt trying to pay for their prescription drugs!

Ninety-one percent of seniors and 61 percent of the rest of us rely on prescription drugs on a regular basis, and these skyrocketing prices are hurting people who don't have prescription-drug insurance, and even those who do. Prescription-drug prices started going up in the 1990s, when they rose 12 percent per year. Around the year 2000, the increases began slowing down, but they're still way out of sync with everything else on the market. Prices for widely used brand-name prescription drugs jumped nearly 9 percent in 2008, according to AARP, which far exceeded the general inflation rate of 3.8 percent. That's how people end up paying $102 a month for a blood-pressure medication called DynaCirc, nearly $200 a month for the sleeping pill Lunesta, and $269 a month to take the antidepressant Cymbalta.

If you think these huge increases don't affect you because you make a good living, or because you don't get sick often, or because you have prescription-drug insurance, think again. First of all, prescription drugs are the great equalizer; they can cost thousands of dollars a year, so unless you're a Rockefeller, paying for them is going to take a painful bite out of your income. Second, even if you don't get sick often, you never know when out of the clear blue sky you'll be diagnosed with a disease that requires you to take drugs that have a whopping price tag—it could be anything from a skin condition to a psychiatric illness to cancer. Third, prescription-drug insurance used to pay for nearly everything, but insurance companies have now shifted much of the cost to us in the form of higher co-payments and deductibles. In 2007, the Patient Advocate Foundation helped more than 44,000 people struggling to pay health-care bills of all kinds, and of all these people 31 percent listed prescription-drug co-payments as their primary financial concern, so you're not safe even if you're wealthy and healthy. It's no wonder, then, that the Center for Studying Health System Change found that between 2003 and 2007 higher-income adults and those without chronic conditions experienced increases in unmet prescription-drug needs that were nearly as large as those with lower incomes and chronic conditions.

SOLUTIONS: HOW TO SAVE MONEY
ON PRESCRIPTION DRUGS

Now let's take a look at how John Bonifield and I solved Bernadine's prescription-drug problem. First, here's a list of what her doctor had prescribed and how much it was costing her:

Zegerid for acid reflux: $154/month
Valtrex for herpes: $197/month
Azor for high blood pressure: $138/month
Bernadine's total monthly prescription-drug bill: $489/month

The trick to helping Bernadine afford her drugs was finding medicines that would work just as well as the ones her doctor prescribed but cost less. By talking to doctors and pharmacists and visiting the Consumer Reports Best Buy Drugs website, we managed to reduce Bernadine's monthly pharmacy bill from $489 to $32 a month! You don't need to be a medical journalist to do this; it's not hard to do the research on your own, and below I explain how. After we aired our story about Bernadine, I received an email from John. "Bernadine saw the segment this morning and called," he said. "She is ecstatic and expresses her thanks to everyone on the team. She said we've restored her hope."

Saving Money on Bernadine's Prescription Drugs

For acid reflux: instead of Zegerid . . . over-the-counter Prilosec
Instead of $154/month . . . $24/month
Bernadine saves $130/month

For herpes: instead of Valtrex . . . generic acyclovir
Instead of $197/month . . . $4/month
Bernadine saves $193/month

For high blood pressure: instead of Azor . . . generic benazepril
Instead of $138/month . . . $4/month
Bernadine saves $134/month

Bernadine's total savings:
Instead of $489/month . . . Bernadine could pay $32/month
Bernadine's total savings: $457/month

> These substitutions won't work for everyone. If you're spending a lot of money on brand-name medicines, ask your doctor if there are less expensive brands, generics, or over-the-counter medicines that will work for you.

So how do you know if there are cheaper alternatives to the drugs your doctor has prescribed? Here's what I call the prescription-drug rule of thumb: *if your disease is common, there's probably a relatively inexpensive drug you can take.* Sometimes they'll be generics, sometimes they'll be over-the-counter drugs, and sometimes they'll be inexpensive brand-name drugs. That's why John and I were able to help Bernadine; herpes, acid reflux, and high blood pressure are all very common diseases. If my friend Lee had known the prescription-drug rule of thumb, she would have thought to herself, Hmm, pregnancy is a common condition, and all pregnant women are supposed to take a prenatal vitamin, so there's got to be a vitamin that's cheaper than $40 a month. After coming to this realization, her first step would have been to ask if her pharmacy had a prenatal vitamin on its $4 generic list. (Also, she could have gone to the pharmacy's website and found the list herself.) I called her pharmacy for her, and indeed it did have a $4 generic prenatal vitamin called Prenatal Plus. Aha! That's ten times less expensive than the drug her doctor prescribed.

It would, of course, have been much less complicated if Lee had simply asked her doctor whether the drug was expensive at the time he wrote the prescription. Unfortunately, she would probably have received a puzzled look in response. That's understandable. Doctors have thousands of patients, and there's no way they can know how much every drug costs in each of our insurance plans (or the pharmacy's charge if we don't have insurance). That's why you have to do what I did for Lee, which is to snoop around on your own and see if there's a less expensive alternative, and then call your doctor (or have your pharmacist call for you) and ask if that cheaper drug would work for you. You should never assume that you absolutely have to have the expensive drug. For example, I asked experts at the American College of Obstetricians and Gynecologists and the March of Dimes whether there was any medical reason that my friend should take the more expensive vitamin. Their answer: no way. "She should call her doctor back and ask if she can take a generic instead, and I bet the answer will be yes," said Dr. Jennifer Niebyl, a spokesperson for the American College of Obstetricians and Gynecologists and a professor of obstetrics and gynecology at the University of Iowa. She explained to me that when it comes down to what's most important in a prenatal vitamin—the folic acid and the iron—there isn't much difference between the expensive brand names and the cheap generics. "The doctor probably has no idea how much this vitamin costs," Dr. Niebyl said. What drugs doctors choose to prescribe is largely based on habit, another obstetrician explained. "Most providers get familiar with one particular brand, and that's what they'll prescribe," said Dr. Diane Ashton, deputy medical director of the March of Dimes. "Some doctors just aren't used to prescribing generics."

I found a $4 generic for Lee, but suppose there hadn't been one. In that case, she could have called her prescription-drug insurance company and asked for the name of the least expensive prenatal vitamin on its list; she could then have called her obstetrician and asked if it was okay for her to take that pill. Now, let's say you don't have prescription-drug insurance. In that case, just call your pharmacy and ask for the least expensive drug that's in the same class as the one your doctor prescribed. If the folks at the pharmacy aren't helpful, go to the Consumer Reports Best Buy Drugs website (crbestbuydrugs.org), which gives the best prices for drugs for various common ailments, such as high cholesterol, depression, and high blood pressure. If you find a drug that costs less than the one your doctor has prescribed, ask him if you can take it.

Having said all this, I totally get it that it may not be easy to tell your doctor that you're looking for cheap drugs. I mean, it's one thing to try to negotiate the price on a used car, but nobody wants to sound cheap when it comes to his health or (even worse) his spouse's or children's health. "We have no idea how to talk about money," says Dr. Vicki Rackner, a surgeon and a patient advocate. "Money is the ultimate taboo." On page 185 of the appendix, I have a sample conversation with a doctor to help you have this touchy (not to mention complicated) discussion about getting cheap drugs.

There's No Such Thing as a Free Lunch . . . or a Free Drug!

When Dr. Richard Adair's internist offered him a free two-week supply of prescription skin cream for his actinic keratosis, Dr. Adair said no thank you. What's wrong with him? Why would anyone say no to free medicine? Dr. Adair, an internist at the University of Minnesota, knew that once he finished the free samples of Aldara, a brand-name drug, he'd have to pay $309.57 for a two-week supply. Fluorouracil, a generic brand that's also used to treat his disease, costs $74.84 for two weeks. Adair went on fluorouracil, and he's been doing great— and saving more than $6,000 a year!

As David Rothman, the director of the Center for the Study of Society and Medicine at the College of Physicians & Surgeons at Columbia University, puts it, "Samples look like they're free, but they're not." Simply put, samples don't last forever. They're usually for the most expensive medicines, and when they run out, you're left paying the price tag. The only situation where it pays to accept a free sample is when it's for a short-term problem, such as an infection. Most samples, however, are for long-term problems, like Dr. Adair's sun-damaged skin, so before accepting a sample, always ask how long you'll need to take the drug.

I must add that, unfortunately, under some circumstances you really are forced to take an expensive drug. For example, if you have certain very serious or rare conditions, there might not be cheaper alternatives. In this case, you can use a Prescription Assistance Plan, programs run by private companies and foundations to help lower costs for patients. Consumer Reports has a guide to choosing the best program; Google "Consumer Reports prescription assistance programs." Another money-saving idea is to split pills under certain circumstances. Let's say, for example, that you need 10 milligrams of a drug that comes in both 10 milligrams and 20 milligrams. You could ask your doctor for a prescription for 20 milligrams and split the pills, doubling your supply. Note: ask your doctor before you do this, and buy a pill-splitting device from a drugstore; don't use a knife. Consumer Reports also offers tips on how to split pills safely; Google "Consumer Reports splitting pills."

In addition to being a smart consumer of prescription drugs, you need to be a smart purchaser of prescription-drug insurance. With health-care reform, more and more of us will be purchasing insurance on the Exchange, a central website listing all available insurance policies divided into "silver," "gold," and "platinum" levels. As you look through the site, keep in mind that some policies cover prescription drugs and others don't; it may be cheaper to buy one that doesn't and get a separate prescription-drug policy. Compare different policies carefully, and remember that just because two policies are "silver" (or "gold" or "platinum"), they don't necessarily offer the same prescription-drug coverage.

CONCLUSION: HAGGLING FOR HEALTH CARE

When my husband and I began dating, we noticed that our boom boxes were identical. (For you young folks, a boom box is a radio-CD player.) We also discovered we'd bought them at the same store and at pretty much the same time. We got to talking, and it turned out he'd paid $100 for his, while I'd paid $200 for mine. How did he do that? Simple—my husband haggled with the store. He walked in with $100, pointed to the boom box he wanted, said that was what he could pay, and he got it for that price. It never dawned on me that you could do that.

I think one reason my husband thought to haggle and I didn't is that I'm American and he's not. The fine art of haggling is lost in this country; except for cars and houses, we don't think to negotiate prices. During the recession of 2008–2009, writing my "Empowered Patient" column really taught me that prices for many things in health care are, well, bendy. You can negotiate how much you pay a doctor for an office visit. If your doctor prescribes an expensive brand-name drug, you don't have to get that drug; you can see if there's a cheaper alternative. When your optometrist prescribes contact lenses, you don't have to buy them from him; you can go online and get them for less. When your insurance company says it won't pay a hospital bill, you can reverse that decision. Once you realize the power you have, you can save serious amounts of money on health care. Bernadine now knows this little piece of truth, as does my friend Lee, and they're both the richer for it.

Final Checklist: How to Save Money on Health-Care Costs

1. **Do your homework before you go for the doctor's appointment.** Often, you'll know what type of drug your doctor is going to prescribe even before you arrive for the appointment. Let's say, for example, you plan to ask your gynecologist for birth-control pills. Before you go for the appointment, see if your pharmacy has a $4 generic birth-control pill. If it doesn't, call your prescription-drug insurance company and get the name of the least expensive birth-control pill that's available to you. If you don't have insurance, call the pharmacy and find out

how much it charges for different brands of pills. Then, when you see your doctor, you can ask if you can take that specific pill.

2. **Ask your pharmacist for help.** If you get hit with sticker shock at the pharmacy, ask the pharmacist to call your doctor's office and inquire whether you can take a less expensive alternative. You could also make the call, but your pharmacist will probably get a quicker response.

3. **Be wary of samples.** Samples are usually for the highest-priced drugs on the market, so once the samples run out you'll be stuck with the price tag. You'll save money in the long run if you get a prescription for a less expensive drug, even if it means you don't get samples and have to pay for it from the very beginning.

4. **If you absolutely have to take an expensive drug, look into a Prescription Assistance Plan.** Consumer Reports has great advice on how to choose one of these plans, which helps you pay the price of pricey drugs. Another idea: see if you can order a dosage that's twice as high (say, 20 milligrams instead of 10 milligrams) and split the pills in half—with your doctor's permission, of course.

CHAPTER EIGHT

Don't Fall for Medical Marketing

After ten days in the neonatal intensive-care unit, the doctors told us we could finally take our daughter Shir home. A rare Atlanta snowstorm loomed, and we wrapped her up in blankets for the car ride home. Pulling into our driveway, I took Shir out of her car seat and carried her inside, my arms hugging her tightly. Behind me, my husband walked in the door with an overstuffed white plastic bag in each hand, full of all the things we would need to take care of our new baby: preemie diapers and thermometers and tiny hats and baby blankets—and a bottle of barbiturates.

Yes, we brought our baby home from the hospital on barbiturates. Hers was Phenobarbital, and it treated her seizures and saved her life. Her days in the NICU were spent fine-tuning the dosage she needed, because with too little Phenobarbital she could have more seizures. Too much, and she'd be too sleepy to eat. Too, too much and she could die. Once they arrived at the right dose for her, the nurses taught us how to measure the red medicine precisely in tiny syringes. We then mixed it with a little breast milk and poured the pink liquid into special bottles the hospital gave us. Shir enthusiastically drank her pink "phenobarb cocktail" every morning and every night. After a week or so we ran out of the medicine the hospital sent us home with, and I made a trip to the pharmacy to fill the prescription.

"That'll be $3.23," the pharmacist said to me as she handed over the bottle.

"Are you sure?" I asked. "That can't be right." I'd never heard of a drug costing $3.23, even with insurance.

"No, that's right," she said. "That's the entire cost of the drug."

"You mean this drug costs $3.23? For this whole bottle? That's the whole price?" I asked incredulously.

"That's right," she answered.

Thank God, I thought to myself. Not because of the money itself—I didn't care about that. I was relieved because a drug that costs $3.23 must be old. It must be old as the hills. Moses must have taken this drug. And old drugs make me very happy.

LINDA AND DINA: WHEN MEDICAL MARKETING IS HAZARDOUS TO YOUR HEALTH

When a doctor prescribes a drug, you assume she's chosen it because it's the very best medicine on the market for you. You figure that all her scientific smarts, training, and experience have gone into selecting the medicine that's most likely to get you better. While this may be true, what your doctor doesn't tell you is that sometimes she chooses a particular drug because a salesperson for that drug took her out for a steak dinner the night before. Pharmaceutical salespeople are ubiquitous in medicine. They bring your doctor free lunches. They invite her to expensive dinners to hear glowing lectures about their products. They may even have paid your doctor as much as $15,000 to give one of those lectures. What your doctor doesn't tell you is that medical marketing is profiting her but hurting you, because all that money, all that food, all those attractive, fun salespeople are clouding her medical judgment.

This explains why I was so happy that Shir's drug was cheap. Its low price tag told me that no cutie-pie sales rep was pushing the neonatologist to prescribe it; reps don't waste their time pushing drugs that cost $3.23. The neonatologist gave it to Shir because she truly believed in it, not because in between bites of filet mignon some pharma rep said to her, "Hey, Doc, how are those phenobarb scrips working out for you?"

I felt good about Shir's drug, but I've interviewed patients who weren't so lucky. Linda Lewis learned the hard way that when a doctor receives money from a company, it can color her medical judgment. Linda, a graduate student in Southern California, has a bad back, and when she went to an orthopedist for her back pain he told her an artificial disk was just what she needed. "He said my back would be better than ever," Linda told me. "I'm thinking, Wow, disk replacement is the best thing since sliced bread."

After the surgery, Linda says she ended up in debilitating pain, could walk only with the assistance of a walker, and had to have a second procedure to correct the first one. "I couldn't take enough drugs for the pain," she told me. "Having that surgery was the worst decision of my life." Only later did Linda learn that her doctor made money from the company that makes the disk. She was livid when she found out that, according to records from the North American Spine Society, her surgeon had accepted several thousand dollars from the company that makes the artificial disk that messed up her back so badly. This amount is minuscule compared to the $8 million two other physicians received from this company— *each*. (Do you think these two doctors, when they recommended the disk to their patients, added, "And oh, by the way, did I mention this company gave me $8 million"?) Once Linda found out about her surgeon's financial link to this company, it made sense to her that he was enthusiastic about the disk while pooh-poohing the many other options available for treating back pain. Linda has since sued her surgeon.

Dina Foster also discovered after the fact that her doctor had financial ties to a drug company. Nine months after her husband,

Tommy, died of kidney cancer, Dina, a retired elementary-school teacher, told me her story in a heartbreaking email. When Tommy was diagnosed in 2005, surgeons in New York removed his kidney and referred him to an oncologist for further care. At their first meeting with the oncologist, Dina says the doctor was very clear about what they should do. "He told us there was no hope except to enroll in a clinical trial for a drug called Sutent," she said. When the doctor turned to leave the room, Dina asked him about a drug for kidney cancer called Interluekin-2, or IL-2, which their daughter had read about on the Internet. "He turned around and said, 'We don't do that here. There's too much risk for too little benefit,' " Dina recalls. (IL-2 is the same drug I mentioned in chapter 5. It makes tumors disappear in a small percentage of patients.) Since this oncologist was world-renowned, and Tommy had such a good experience with the surgeon at the same hospital, he joined the clinical trial on Sutent without investigating IL-2 or any other drug.

Dina now regrets that decision, as Sutent didn't work for Tommy. His cancer spread, and he died three years later at the age of sixty-five. In her email to me, Dina said she'll forever wonder if her husband might have been better off with the IL-2, if he might have been one of the few patients for whom it worked beautifully. She knows IL-2 is highly toxic and doesn't work for everyone, but she wishes the oncologist had at least given her husband the option of taking it. "At no time was Interleukin ever offered as a choice," she wrote to me in an email. "I will always wonder if things would have been different if we had had the Interleukin in the beginning. I know it is a risky procedure, but Tommy might have been one of the 8 to 10 percent who responded. I think we should have been given the choice."

I talked this over with Dr. James Yang, a senior investigator at the National Cancer Institute and an expert on kidney cancer, who said it was clear to him that both Sutent and IL-2 should have been discussed with Dina and Tommy. "I think the real failing is to not present all options in a balanced and non-biased way," Dr. Yang says.

Only later did Dina find out that her husband's oncologist had financial ties to the company that makes Sutent. Financial-disclosure statements filed with the American Society of Clinical Oncology and included in this doctor's journal articles confirm his financial relationship with Pfizer, which makes the drug. The way Dina sees it, Sutent was this doctor's "baby." Dina's conclusion: "If a doctor's taking money from a drug company, he's going to push that drug. I think there were injustices done to my husband."

WHAT THE STUDIES SAY

Relationships between doctors and the pharmaceutical industry "begin in medical school, continue during residency training, and persist throughout physicians' careers," writes Dr. David Blumenthal, the former director of the Institute for Health Policy at Harvard Medical School, who later went on to work in the Obama administration. Drug companies invest heavily in these relationships, employing 90,000 salespeople, or one salesperson for every five office-based physicians. In a 2007 study, researchers at Harvard reported that 94 percent of doctors acknowledged having some type of relationship with pharmaceutical companies, whether it was getting free lunches or lucrative speaking engagements or funding to enroll patients in the company's drug trials. Another study showed that the average doctor meets with drug reps four times a month, and many physicians see drug reps in their offices every day. There's so much money at stake—in 2007 Americans spent $287 million on prescription drugs—it's no wonder drug companies do everything they can to get doctors to prescribe their products. Those millions of dollars are why "a battle is being waged to win the hearts and minds of the physicians who write 2.2 billion drug prescriptions annually in the United States," as one doctor put it.

Here's a legitimate question: Who cares if my doctor takes a free lunch from a drug company every now and then? I mean, he's a big boy, right? He's smart enough not to be influenced by an occasional sandwich. My doctor uses medical facts, not marketing data, to decide which drugs to prescribe for me, right? Studies would disagree with you. One study, which looked at twenty-nine other studies, found that when a doctor met with a pharmaceutical rep his rates for prescribing that company's drug went up. A financial analysis done for the pharmaceutical industry by researchers at Yale University found that for every dollar the industry invested in marketing top-selling drugs, the company made $10.60 in sales.

This makes perfect sense. Pharmaceutical companies aren't dumb. There's a reason they spend $12 billion a year marketing to physicians. Marketing to physicians is obviously effective, "otherwise, why would the pharmaceutical industry spend $30,000 annually on each and every one of us?" Drs. Mark Mahowald and Michel Cramer Bornemann asked in an article in the medical journal *Sleep Medicine*.

Former drug-company salespeople tell me they don't need studies to convince them that marketing gets doctors to prescribe certain drugs; they experienced this firsthand, because pharmaceutical companies have access to databases that allow them to track an individual doctor's prescriptions down to the last pill. "The industry only does things that show a return on investment," says Kathleen Slattery-Moschkau, who was a drug rep for ten years. "So let's say I took Dr. Smith to L'Etoile, an expensive French restaurant. I would look at his prescriptions two weeks later and I would be able to see if I'd had an impact on his sales." If the L'Etoile dinner didn't work, she'd try something else. There was nothing mysterious about any of this: it was all there in black and white in the doctor's prescription record.

Jamie Reidy, another former drug rep and the author of *Hard Sell: The Evolution of a Viagra Salesman,* has a phrase for this—he calls it "circling the day." On his calendar he'd circle the day on which he did something for a doctor, such as taking him out to dinner, and later he'd check his sales figures to see if the doctor had increased his prescription. He told me about one particularly successful circled day. "I was selling a drug called Cardura for frequent urination. Our big competition was a drug called Flomax. I was trying to learn more about these two big urologists in town, so I asked their staff about all the standard men things: Do they like cigars? Baseball? Golf? But none of these things appealed. Then one of the nurses told me the doctors loved to fish, and they hadn't been fishing in forever. Bing! I took these two urologists fly-fishing on the American River. We drove out the night before, so I paid for their hotels and a steak dinner. Early the next morning, we had our own boat and private guides. It was off the charts. I had to leave these guys on the river in the middle of the day because I had a hot date in San Francisco, and as I was leaving I turned to them and said, 'Did the Flomax guy ever treat you like this?' One of the urologists yelled back, 'What Flomax?' " Reidy checked the two doctors' sales when the numbers came in a few weeks later. They had skyrocketed. Both doctors went from prescribing Cardura hardly at all to writing more than ten prescriptions a week.

Reidy told me about another scheme he used to get doctors to prescribe his drug. As a sales rep for Pfizer, he was having zero success getting a certain physician to prescribe Pfizer's latest antibiotic, Trovan. Every time Reidy received his sales reports, he'd scan the column looking for Dr. Reluctant's sales figures, and every time he'd see a big fat zero. Reidy didn't know what to do. Why couldn't he get this doctor to prescribe Trovan? He'd worked so hard, charming the office manager, flirting with the doctor's nurses, bringing flowers to the secretaries. Reidy had used these tactics with great success in the past, but they weren't working with Dr. Reluctant.

On his next visit to sell drugs to Dr. Reluctant, Reidy went through his usual routine: he walked into this doctor's office, chatted up the secretaries, and hoped to be invited into the back office, where he might be able to persuade the nurses to get him a private audience with Dr. Reluctant. If his boyish charm didn't work with the nurses, he knew what would. "My research found chocolate to be the best motivator for female office staff members," he wrote in *Hard Sell*. "Consequently, I became the 'M&M's guy.'" And the chocolate worked—he saw drug sales go up.

The back office has another advantage for an enterprising drug rep: once there, he or she can search for clues about a doctor's personal life. "Our training in sales school is akin to the training they give in spy agencies, like the CIA," says Shahram Ahari, who sold drugs in New York City for Eli Lilly in the late 1990s, the same time Reidy was "carrying the bag" for Pfizer in Indiana and California. "Reps scour a doctor's office for objects—a tennis racquet, Russian novels, seventies rock music, fashion magazines, travel mementos, or cultural or religious symbols—that can be used to establish a personal connection with the doctor," Ahari wrote in an article that he co-authored in a medical journal. "We were taught to soak up everything in the environment. So we'd learn that Dr. So-and-So was gay and lives downtown with his boyfriend and that this other doctor has two kids named Jimmy and Susie and their birthdays are March 1 and July 23." Reps were trained to commit these kinds of details to memory long enough to get back to the car, where they'd immediately type them into their laptops so that at the next visit they could be sure to remember to ask about the doctor's vacation in Florida or the outcome of little Jimmy's soccer game. The details about the doctors would go into the drug company's central database so other reps in the company who sold drugs to the same doctor could also see them. "We compiled dossiers on each doctor," Ahari explained to me.

Back to Reidy and Dr. Reluctant. So far, all the sleuthing in the world hadn't revealed anything that might get Dr. Reluctant to start writing prescriptions for Trovan. But on this trip Reidy got lucky. He overheard the doctor mention to one of his nurses that his father had terrible allergies. Reidy told me, "He just said it in passing, but I jumped on it. I told him, 'Hold on, I'll be right back.' I ran out into the parking lot, hopped in my car, and called a friend of mine I knew from the days when I sold Zyrtec. I jumped onto the highway, drove for about an hour, got a bunch of Zyrtec samples, and came back. I handed them to the doctor to give to his father. The doctor took them and turned to his nurse and said, 'Everyone gets Trovan from now on.'"

Two weeks later, when Reidy received his sales numbers, he went directly to the Trovan section. "His numbers went through the roof!" Reidy recalls. Dr. Reluctant went from writing no prescriptions at all for Trovan to writing more than ten prescriptions a week. "I was elated. I actually voice-mailed my boss and said, 'I'm making it happen!'

"And then," Reidy told me, "Trovan made people's livers blow up."

Huh?

A few months after Reidy's quick thinking and fast driving persuaded a doctor to start prescribing Trovan in spades, the Food and Drug Administration issued a warning about reports of rare but sometimes deadly liver problems among people taking Trovan. Pfizer agreed to start distributing Trovan solely to hospitals and nursing homes, where patients could be closely monitored, and where doctors were warned to use the drug only under extremely limited circumstances. That meant the end of the Trovan business for Jamie Reidy.

Trovan certainly looked safe when it came on the market in

1998. None of the 7,000 patients who took it in premarketing clinical trials had the liver problems that later killed people. But as time went on and millions of people began taking Trovan, the liver problems started showing up. The sad thing is that some of these people with trashed livers perhaps didn't even need to be on Trovan; an older antibiotic, one with a longer safety record, might have worked just as well. There's an excellent chance that these patients were taking Trovan not because it was necessarily better for them but because a clever rep like Reidy had learned the exact button to push with their doctors: the right restaurant for dinner, the right lunch to bring into the office, or a batch of Zyrtec for a doctor's allergy-prone father.

Trovan is hardly the only new drug that was pushed with wild enthusiasm only to be reined back in later because of safety concerns. Remember the fen-phen craze in the late 1990s? Doctors at the Mayo Clinic discovered that one of the drugs in fen-phen might be causing heart-valve problems, and it was taken off the market. Then there's the antibiotic Raxar, which was pushed by drug reps—until doctors discovered it might cause a potentially fatal irregular heartbeat and it was taken off the shelves. The heart drug Posicor went belly-up after less than a year on the market because it reacted badly with twenty-six other drugs. And, of course, who can forget Vioxx? It was approved in 1999 and, in all my years as a medical correspondent, seldom have I seen a drug come out with such fanfare. It was as if this pain reliever were going to cure cancer. Doctors' offices were thick with reps touting its benefits, and the marketing clearly worked: Vioxx was prescribed for 84 million people. But as drug reps were pushing Vioxx, it became clear that people taking this wildly popular drug were more likely to suffer from heart attacks and strokes. In 2004, Merck pulled Vioxx off the market. Years later, the lawsuits continue.

This is why I was relieved to find out Shir was taking an old drug. By the time Shir began taking Phenobarbital, it had been used for ninety-two years, and after ninety-two years doctors are aware of the side effects, unlike with the brand-spanking-new drugs described above. After ninety-two years, there are seldom surprises, and that's exactly what we wanted for our precious baby. Old drugs, when they work as well as new drugs, are a win-win for the patient; they have a longer tried-and-true safety record, and they're prescribed because they work, not because they've been marketed heavily.

Now, you might be thinking that even if drug reps are influencing your doctor, this isn't necessarily a bad thing. After all, these reps are educated scientists, passing along medical wisdom to your doctor, right? That's what Shahram Ahari used to think. Ahari became a drug rep fresh out of college, with a degree in biochemistry and molecular biology. When he reported for sales training, he found that he was unique. "I was part of Lilly's elite neuroscience team," he told me. "There were twenty-one of us, and I was the only one with college-level science training." When Ahari graduated from sales school, he was determined to sell his drugs based on their medical benefits. "I thought I'd be debating the merits of drugs with doctors in the language of hard science," he told me. But the scientific approach failed; his sales numbers were dismal. "Then I'd take them out for a $700 dinner in the city and we'd see a massive spike," he said. Here's another thing that told Ahari science didn't really matter. "We gave them an 800 number manned by MDs and PharmDs. The doctors could call and discuss scientific questions and have material faxed, emailed, or mailed to them. I saw two hundred doctors a month, and maybe one of them would use this service," he said.

Former rep Jamie Reidy's only college science class was Chemistry 101, which he had to drop because he was failing it. He told me, "Every day [as a sales rep] I thought to myself, 'Who am I and what am I doing here? What's wrong with you people and why are you listening to me?'" Gene Carbona started working as a drug rep ten days after graduating from college with a degree in political science. He told me, "I'd call my mom and dad and say, 'I talked to cardiovascular surgeons today and I made them change their minds about what they were prescribing for chronic obstructive pulmonary disorder!' My parents would say, 'Isn't that against the law?' and I'd say, 'No, that's what my company trained me to do. We're trained to get doctors to use the newest, most expensive drugs we have.' "

After many years in the industry, Kathleen Slattery-Moschkau, who also had no training in science before she became a sales rep, began to worry she'd become a little too good at getting doctors to do what she wanted. "I left the industry for a lot of reasons, but one was that something I said, or didn't say, to a physician was going to hurt someone," she told me. "I couldn't sleep at night. Our jobs had nothing to do with truly educating doctors. It was all about how to get a doctor to write a prescription."

SOLUTIONS: HOW TO MAKE SURE YOU'RE GETTING THE DRUGS THAT ARE BEST FOR YOU

Gene Carbona is a bit of an in-your-face kind of guy. When his internist handed him a prescription for an expensive antibiotic for pink eye, he exploded. "I looked at it and said, 'Are you out of your mind? You're prescribing me an antibiotic that's $7.50 per pill when you could be writing me a prescription for an antibiotic that's eleven cents a pill?' " Carbona, a former pharmaceutical rep who now works for an independent website that evaluates drugs, pulled up the data on his Palm Pilot. "I showed her how the eleven-cent pill worked just as well as the $7.50 pill."

Here's where I would have loved to have been a fly on the wall.

"I told her, 'I walk by your office every day on my way to get pizza, and I see that every day the drug reps bring lunch for your office.' She tells me, 'Gene, I really didn't write you that drug because of all that . . . but maybe I did.' " The doctor then handed Gene a prescription for the cheaper drug.

"I have a wonderful primary-care physician," Gene tells me. "She's the smartest woman who went to the best medical school and got the best grades. But boy does she love her drug reps."

We all want to make sure we're getting the best drugs with the longest safety record, but I know I'm not quite as bold as Gene. I couldn't just confront a doctor the way he did. If you're like me, you might do what I did when I found myself in a situation similar to Gene's with his pink eye. When I first moved to Atlanta in the 1990s, I ran out of my prescription allergy medicine. I went to a local allergist to get a prescription for my nasal spray, and here's the conversation that ensued:

ME: I've had ragweed allergies for many years, and a prescription nasal spray, Beconase, works really well for me. Could you prescribe it for me, please?

DR. SNEEZE: Beconase is an old drug. How about Flonase? I think you ought to try that instead.

ME (*noting the Flonase pen in the doctor's hand*): I really like Beconase. I feel great, and there are no side effects. Why would this one be better?

DR. SNEEZE: Because it's newer. Just came out. Better formulation.

ME (*noting the Flonase notepad on his desk*): What, exactly, is better about it? I really love Beconase.

DR. SNEEZE: Flonase is just better. Newer. But if you want the Beconase, I'll give it to you.

ME (*noting the Flonase pamphlets on his shelf*): Thank you, Doctor.

This incident took place back in the nineties, and it's not as easy now as it was then to notice drug paraphernalia in doctors' offices. That's because in 2009, after much pressure from consumer advocates and Congress, the drug industry decided to police itself and stop giving out tchotchkes like pens, notepads, and mugs to doctors. Now you have to sleuth around a bit more to detect whether a pharma rep has been visiting your doctor and possibly influencing her choice of what drug to give you. Check to see if there are pamphlets lying around, or anatomical models on the shelves from certain drug companies—the pharmaceutical industry considers these "educational items" and, unlike the mugs and pens, they're still allowed. After you look for these things, keep an eye out in the waiting room and hallways for a certain type of person. "If you see an extremely attractive, impeccably dressed, polite person with a briefcase in the waiting room, watch out! That's most likely a drug rep," advises Dr. Daniel Carlat, an assistant clinical professor of psychiatry at Tufts University School of Medicine who blogs about the industry's influence on physicians.

While you walk from the waiting room to the examining room, try to sneak a peek into the break room and see if the staff is eating a catered meal. Drug reps love to influence with food, and that's still allowed under the new rules. What better way to get some time with doctors and nurses than to feed them? But perhaps the best way to tell if your doctor has been visited by a drug rep is when the doctor offers you a sample of a drug. These samples aren't left by the drug fairy; they're left by pharmaceutical reps, who know doctors love them and are more likely to prescribe a drug that's in their sample closet than one that isn't. For this reason, one former rep described samples as "pharmaceutical crack."

Even in the absence of cute reps, lunches, and samples, you can still detect if your doctor is under the influence of the pharmaceutical industry. You'll have to be clever, like my friend Tori. When Tori suffered painful uterine bleeding, she went to the gynecologist's office, where the nurse met with her first and encouraged her to have a procedure using a new tool, a wand that would be inserted through the vagina and the cervix, applying electromagnetic energy to remove the lining of her uterus in an effort to stop the bleeding.

But the nurse did her job just a little too well. "She was so positive about it, I thought it was unnatural," Tori told me. "No one should be that thrilled about one option. My visceral reaction was, This doesn't feel right."

When Tori saw the gynecologist, she asked for other ways to treat uterine bleeding besides the wand. It turned out that there were several other approaches, and Tori went with a surgical procedure that's been around forever and for which there are no reps because no special tools are required. "I wanted to go with the tried and true," she told me.

Tori says it's absolutely possible that this new wand, which has been heavily marketed by the company that makes it, would have worked for her. It just made her nervous that the nurse was so enthusiastic about it; she felt that perhaps the judgment of the entire office had been clouded by whatever rep had been there pushing it. She was also nervous about something that was so new.

Unbridled enthusiasm for one medical option over another can be a very bad sign. Years ago, I called a prominent psychiatrist for a story about postpartum depression because he was considered to be one of the leaders—if not *the* leader—in the field. On the phone with me he was adamant about two things: nearly all women with postpartum depression needed antidepressants, and the best choice for them was clearly the drug Effexor. I asked him if there might be other approaches for women with postpartum depression, but he seemed really set on Effexor. After we hung up, I decided not to use his quotes in my story. I knew many other journalists had quoted him, and that he was highly respected, but there was just something about him that seemed so, well, unbelievable. How could every woman with postpartum depression need the same drug? Years later, I was grateful I'd made that decision. This psychiatrist was removed from his post as chairman of his university's psychiatry department and eventually left the university after it was discovered he'd accepted money from drug companies and failed to report it. Much of the money came from Wyeth Pharmaceuticals, which makes Effexor.

This got me to thinking: how would this doctor's patients have known about his financial relationship to drug companies, especially Wyeth? First of all, you can use your intuition, as Tori and I did, and question recommendations (or at least eye them skeptically) when you feel that someone is enthusiastically pushing one approach unequivocally above all others. If there are several treatments for an illness (as there are for many diseases) and your doctor seems absolutely sold on just one of them, it's time to start being skeptical. If your instincts say something is amiss, you can see if the doctor has written any articles about your disease. These days, most medical journals require their authors to reveal whether they've received any money from drug companies or similar groups. Use Google Scholar or PubMed to find the articles, and look for the financial-disclosure section, which is usually at the end of the abstract (the summary that appears at the beginning of the study), or at the very end of the study. You can also find out about a doctor's financial ties by looking up presentations she might have given at medical conferences. Find the major conference associated with her specialty—for example, the American Society of Clinical Oncology for cancer docs or the American College of Cardiology for cardiologists. Search for her name and you'll see if she had to disclose any financial conflicts of interest when she spoke at a conference.

You can also just ask your doctor if she has any financial ties to a drug or device company. This will probably feel uncomfortable. No one wants to appear to be questioning a doctor's (or anyone's) ethics. You could try phrasing it like this: "Doctor, forgive me for asking, but I routinely ask this of all my physicians. Do you have a financial relationship with any drug companies?" or "Doctor, you're prescribing Drug X. Do you have any affiliation with the company that makes it?" If the answer is "Yes," this doesn't mean your doctor's advice is absolutely unreliable, it just means that you should keep this financial relationship with the drug company in mind when considering her advice to take a certain drug or use a particular device.

CONCLUSION: FOLLOW THE MONEY

The rules have changed since the days when Jamie Reidy, Gene Carbona, Shahram Ahari, and Kathleen Slattery-Moschkau pushed prescription drugs. Reidy says if he were a drug rep now, his little fly-fishing expedition, for example, wouldn't fly, since in 2009 the pharmaceutical industry, as part of its overall marketing changes, nixed purely recreational outings between drug salesmen and physicians. These are guidelines only, however, and don't have the force of law. Several former reps I talked to said they still have friends in the industry, and they've heard that these outings continue despite the new rules. "U2 is coming to town, and my friend [a drug rep] already bought tickets for doctors and pharmacists," Gene Carbona told me. "This happens every day of the week."

I don't know for sure if that's true, but I do know that even without the fly-fishing expeditions or the free tickets to Broadway shows, pharmaceutical and drug-device reps still have plenty of ways of influencing doctors to use their products. They can still buy lunch for the staff. They can still pay for doctors' meals when they come to listen to another doctor talk about the benefits of a drug. And the doctor who's doing the speaking—she's paid a consulting fee and can have her travel, lodging, and meal expenses paid for by the company. While some doctors have rejected interaction of any kind with pharmaceutical reps, they remain a minority. For those who do still accept overtures from drug companies you have to ask yourself the question posed by Eric Campbell, an associate professor of health policy at Harvard Medical School: "Let's say your investment counselor went on a trip to Aruba, paid for by a certain company. Then he comes home and recommends that you invest in that company. Wouldn't you be concerned?"

Final Checklist: How to Make Sure Your Doctor Is Prescribing the Drug That Is Best for You

1. **If you know an old, cheap drug works well for you, don't let your doctor talk you into taking a new, more expensive one.** Learn from my nasal-spray experience: if an old drug works for you, don't let your doctor talk you into using something new and shiny unless there's a very specific and compelling reason. Newer drugs have less of a track record and are more expensive.

2. **Try to figure out whether drug reps have been influencing your doctor.** Look around the waiting room to see if there are any young, well-dressed attractive people with rolling suitcases. They're probably drug reps. If there are pamphlets from drug companies lying around, or anatomical models on the shelves from drug companies, that means reps have been there. Ditto for drug samples or catered meals in the break room.

3. **Be wary of a doctor's or nurse's enthusiasm for one drug or surgical approach.** If a doctor or a nurse pushes one drug or surgical device, ask if there are other options. If she says there are none, do your own research to make sure she's right. If she says there are other options, don't let her just write them off; make sure she explains why the option she's pushing is truly the best one for you.

4. **If your doctor is partial to one option, see if she has a financial interest in it.** Do your own research: go on the Internet to look up medical journal articles and conference presentations and see if your doctor has received money from the company that makes the drug or device in question.

5. **Ask your doctor if she has a financial interest in the drug**

or device she has suggested for you. No one wants to appear to be questioning a doctor's (or anyone's) ethics, so this will probably be uncomfortable. You could try phrasing your question like this: "Doctor, forgive me for asking, but I routinely ask this of all my physicians. Do you have a financial relationship with any drug companies?" or "Doctor, you're prescribing Drug X. Do you have any affiliation with the company that makes it?"

CHAPTER NINE

Don't Let a Hospital Kill You

A t the end of a day of downhill skiing deep in the Sierra Nevada, Chuck Toeniskoetter, a commercial building developer, suffered a severe stroke that paralyzed his right side. He says he's alive today because of a nurse and a paramedic who thought quickly, and argued hard, at the top of a snowy mountain.

Someone called a helicopter ambulance, and the nurse and the paramedic, who worked at the resort, urged the pilot to go to Sutter Roseville Medical Center, a certified stroke center, where Chuck could get a lifesaving, clot-busting drug called tPA. The pilot, however, insisted on taking Chuck to a hospital that was fifteen minutes closer, which wasn't a stroke center and wouldn't have tPA. The nurse and the paramedic pleaded with the pilot to go to Sutter, but the pilot stood firm, arguing that the closest hospital was the better option. Finally, the paramedic actually clung to the helicopter door to make sure the pilot didn't take off, and the pilot relented. Chuck was flown to Sutter, where he received tPA, the only drug approved by the Food and Drug Administration to treat ischemic strokes. The drug, which breaks up the blood clots that cause a stroke, can significantly reverse the effects of stroke and reduce the chances of permanent disability *provided it's administered within three hours of the start of stroke symptoms.* Chuck arrived just within that deadline, and he fully recovered. Today, you would never know that he had had a stroke.

Chuck calls those extra fifteen minutes he spent in the ambulance going to Sutter "the shortest fifteen minutes of my life," because they got him to the right hospital. He'll be forever grateful to the nurse and the paramedic who made sure the pilot went to a hospital that administered tPA. "They stood on the runners of the helicopter and were relentless with the pilot," Chuck recalls. "They saved my life."

DENNIS QUAID: SAVING OTHERS FROM HOSPITAL MISTAKES

What your doctor doesn't tell you is that while the right hospital can save you, the wrong hospital can kill you. Sometimes patients die because they end up in the wrong hospital for their particular ailment, which almost happened to Chuck. At other times, emergency rooms move too slowly to help a dying patient. Sometimes—sadly, tens of thousands of times a year—hospitals kill patients by giving them deadly infections. And there are times when hospital workers make mistakes that kill patients. It's frightening to think about, because we trust hospitals to take care of us when we're at our most vulnerable, but there's no question that they can be very scary places.

The actor Dennis Quaid never gave much thought to the dangers lurking in hospitals. He'd been in hospitals before, once for a hernia operation for himself and once when his oldest son was born, and he just assumed that hospitals did everything they could to make sure no one got hurt. Quaid's a pilot—he flies jets—and knows that in aviation you check and double-check everything, and he figured hospitals did the same. But when his twins were born he discovered that hospitals don't double-check everything. In fact, sometimes they don't even check once.

Life for Thomas Boone and Zoe Grace Quaid started out normally. They were born healthy, but a few days after leaving the hospital their parents noticed that Thomas—or T-Boone, as they call him—had red spots under the remnants of his umbilical cord, and that both T-Boone's and Zoe Grace's fingers were turning yellow. Their pediatrician suspected a *Staphylococcus* bacterial infection and told Quaid and his wife, Kimberly, to take the babies to Cedars-Sinai Medical Center for a course of treatment with intravenous antibiotics. In the hospital, the Quaids were truly involved, empowered patients, asking questions constantly about their children's care. For example, Quaid remembers asking about a medicine the nurse was putting into the babies' IV lines. She explained that the drug would flush out the IV so that it wouldn't clog up. At the time, that answer satisfied Dennis.

Now he wishes he had been even more vigilant.

One night as the Quaids were getting ready to go home, they asked the nurses to call them if anything changed. At 7:30 P.M., they called from home to check on the babies, and the nurses reported that everything was fine. Then, at 9 P.M., Kimberly was hit with an overwhelming sense of dread. "The babies are passing," she cried out inconsolably. To reassure his wife, Dennis called the hospital again, and again the nurse told him the babies were perfectly okay. The Quaids finally fell into a fitful sleep.

When they went to the hospital the next morning to visit T-Boone and Zoe Grace, the head nurse and a hospital executive met them at the door to the babies' room. They took the Quaids aside and explained to them that a terrible mistake had been made: their babies had received a huge overdose of a blood-thinning medication called heparin. They were bleeding uncontrollably, and doctors were desperately trying to save their lives. "It was the beginning of the most frightening day of our lives," Quaid testified six months later to a congressional committee holding a hearing about medication errors. "[The babies] were fighting for their lives. Their now water-thin blood was flowing out of every place that they had been poked or prodded. They faced the very real possibility of hemorrhaging through a vein or artery, causing massive brain damage or failure of one of their vital organs." As a nurse tried to stop the bleeding from T-Boone's umbilical cord, it squirted six feet into the air and spattered all over the wall. "They were both screaming in pain, and God only knows what they were feeling. I am not sure even a lab rat had ever received such a high dose of the heparin that was causing them to bleed out," Quaid testified.

The doctors finally managed to control the bleeding and, thankfully, the Quaid twins made a full recovery. But Dennis Quaid learned an important lesson. "Now I know," he told me, "how dangerous a hospital can really be."

An investigation by Cedars-Sinai showed that the babies were supposed to receive a drug called Hep-Lock to flush out the IV lines and prevent clotting. But instead they were given heparin, which is the same medicine but a thousand times stronger. The babies had received this horrific overdose not just once but twice. How could such a grave error happen in one of the best hospitals in the country? Cedars-Sinai later explained that a series of "preventable errors" caused the nurse to administer the wrong medicine. First, the pharmacy technician sent the higher-dose heparin (10,000 units per milliliter) instead of the lower-dose medicine (10 units per milliliter) to the pediatric pharmacy. Then a technician in the pediatric pharmacy failed to verify the concentration, and the higher-dose heparin was delivered to the location in the pediatrics unit where the lower-dose heparin is usually kept. The nurse grabbed the bottle without checking to make sure it was the right concentration and gave it to the babies. It certainly didn't help that the labels for the two drugs were extremely similar. In fact, if the bottles are rotated and the labels are partially hidden from view, which often happens during storage, the two drugs are virtually indistinguishable.

The thing that probably horrifies me the most about this error is that Cedars-Sinai wasn't the first to make it. The same heparin mistake occurred many times before that fateful day in 2007 when the Quaid twins were overdosed, and it's happened since. For example, in 2006, three infants died after an Indianapolis hospital gave them an overdose of heparin. In 2008, fourteen infants were overdosed with heparin at a Corpus Christi, Texas, hospital. Why were these hospitals even using heparin to flush out IV lines? For many years, safety advocates had been urging hospitals to use saline instead, which is much safer. Cedars-Sinai switched to saline (and made other safety changes) only after the publicity surrounding the mistake with the Quaid twins.

The Quaids could have left the entire incident behind them, but because they wanted to protect other families, Dennis Quaid speaks publicly about what patients must do to avoid being the victims of a medication mistake at a hospital. The first step is to be there with your loved one in the hospital, but even that's not enough. "The first overdose occurred right under my nose," Quaid noted when we talked. You also have to ask the right questions. To find out what Quaid wishes he had asked in the hospital, see the box below.

Quaid says he owes it to his children to go on this mission to make hospitals safer and patients more aware. "We're trying to make lemonade out of lemons," he says. "These two little guys went through an ordeal, and now they're going to change the world."

Dennis Quaid's Tips for Keeping Safe in the Hospital

Here are five basic questions Dennis Quaid and hospital safety experts advise all hospital patients to ask.

1. **Is this medicine meant for someone else?** Patients sometimes get medicine that was intended for another patient. When you or a loved one is a patient in a hospital, ask the nurse to verify that a drug really is meant for you, and double-check it yourself by looking at the medication label and making sure that it has the right name on it.

2. **Is this the right drug?** Ask the nurse the name of the medication, and double-check it yourself by looking at the label.

3. **Is this the right dose?** Ask the nurse to tell you the dosage you're supposed to receive (how many milliliters or grams, etc.), then check the label to make sure the dosage is correct.

4. **Is this the right route?** Drugs can be delivered in several ways, including by mouth, in a shot, or through an intravenous line. Ask whether the medication you're about to get is supposed to be given to you in the way it's being given.

5. **Is this the right time?** Medications are supposed to be given at a certain frequency: twice a day, once every four hours, etc. Ask the nurse how often the drug is supposed to be given, and when was the last time you received it.

WHAT THE STUDIES SAY

"We were lucky we had a happy ending," Dennis Quaid told me. He knows that every year in the United States as many as 98,000 people die in hospitals because of preventable medication errors, according to a study by the Institute of Medicine. These hospital mistakes kill more people than car accidents, breast cancer, or AIDS. According to another IOM report, at least one medication error will happen to you *every single day* that you spend in the hospital. "It's like a major airline crash every day of every year," Quaid says. "It's outrageous. When an airplane crashes, it's big news all over television. But with medical errors there's kind of a conspiracy of silence. What happened to my children did make news only because I'm a prominent person." The important message for all of us is to be aware that hospital errors are not unusual. As *60 Minutes* noted when Quaid was interviewed on the program, "If it can happen to the children of a movie star, at one of the finest hospitals in the country, it can happen to anyone."

In addition to the 98,000 people who are killed by medication errors in hospitals, another 99,000 Americans die each year from infections they acquire in the hospital, according to the Centers for Disease Control and Prevention. These patients are admitted to the hospital free of infection, catch an infection *from* the hospital, and come out in a casket. Approximately one out of every twenty-two patients who checks into a U.S. hospital acquires a bacterial infection, adding more than $28 billion to health-care costs, according to a 2009 report from the CDC. These figures aren't particularly surprising, considering the lousy job many health-care workers do when it comes to washing their hands. The CDC says health-care workers have a "poor" record of following very basic hand-washing procedures, with only 40 percent adhering to recommended guidelines.

Errors and infections aren't the only dangers lurking in hospitals. While emergency rooms generally do an excellent job of saving lives, long waits are an issue. This came to national attention in 2007, when Edith Rodriguez lay on the floor of a Los Angeles hospital emergency room vomiting blood, and witnesses say no one did anything to help her. Her boyfriend actually called 911 from the hospital and was refused help because they were already in a hospital. ("It's not an emergency. It is not an emergency," the 911 operator said on tape.) Rodriguez died in the ER of a perforated bowel.

According to one report, in 2008 the average total waiting time in a U.S. emergency room was four hours and three minutes, a twenty-seven-minute increase in nationwide average wait times since 2002—that's a big jump in just six years. A 2008 Harvard study of more than 90,000 U.S. emergency-room visits found that one in four heart-attack patients waited fifty minutes or more to be seen by a physician in the ER. "Ridiculously long wait times are a huge issue," Dr. David Beiser, an ER physician at the University of Chicago Medical Center, told me. "Recently we've had over forty patients in our waiting room. When I was in training (five years ago), it was rare to see more than twenty patients in our waiting room."

Finally, as Chuck Toeniskoetter learned, a hospital can also kill you if it's not suited to respond to your particular medical situation. Whether it's a stroke, a high-risk birth, or a heart attack, studies show it's worth doing whatever it takes to get to a hospital that has the right equipment and staff with the best training. For example, a study in the *Archives of Internal Medicine* shows that heart-attack patients have a higher chance of surviving if they're brought to one of *U.S. News & World Report*'s top 50 hospitals for treating heart problems. Another study, this one in *The New England Journal of Medicine,* finds that very low-birthweight newborns are more likely to survive if treated in a high-level neonatal intensive-care unit that takes care of a large volume of very low-birthweight babies. "A lot of people think hospitals are all the same," said Dr. Samantha Collier, the chief medical officer at HealthGrades, which ranks hospitals. "They're not."

SOLUTIONS: HOW TO STAY SAFE IN THE HOSPITAL

In this chapter I'll tell you how to do your best to avoid the four big dangers lurking in hospitals: you choose the wrong hospital (the problem Chuck almost had); you don't get the care you need in the emergency room (Edith Rodriguez's downfall); you become the victim of a medical error (the plight of the Quaid twins); and you get an infection from the hospital (I'll tell you more about Josh Nahum, a young man who died from a bacteria that he picked up while he was in the hospital).

CHOOSING THE RIGHT HOSPITAL

First, let's talk about choosing the right hospital from the get-go. Of course, sometimes in an emergency you have no choice where to go, but if you know that you have a particular medical condition, you can think ahead about what would be the best possible hospital for you if something should go wrong. For example, when I was pregnant with babies two, three, and four, I knew that I stood a pretty good chance of having a premature baby, because I had a history of preeclampsia. In the back of my mind, I always knew which hospitals in Atlanta had Level III neonatal intensive-care units (that's the highest level), and when I traveled I checked beforehand to see where the Level III NICUs in that city were located. If someone in your family has a heart condition, you can go on websites (I'll give you a list in a minute) and find the best cardiac-care hospitals in your area so you'll know where he should go in case of an emergency; as we saw from the study I mentioned earlier, you've got a better chance of surviving a heart attack if you're in a hospital that has a good cardiac program. If you have children, you pretty much know that at some point you're going to end up in the emergency room with some ailment or injury. Check to see if there are children's hospitals in your area; while all ERs take care of kids, children's hospitals are specially equipped to do so, and under certain circumstances it might be worth the extra time to go there.

Before you have a scheduled procedure, invest time in learning about which hospitals have a good track record for that procedure. "If we're going to spend hours on the Internet doing research before we buy a car, we should spend at least as much time researching hospitals," Dr. Collier says. To find out which hospitals rank highest for certain specialties, you can go to www.healthgrades.com or www.leapfroggroup.org. On these sites you can find out, say, the best place to get hip surgery in Topeka, Kansas, or the best place to have a premature baby in New York City. Here are some other useful sites for choosing a hospital: the Joint Commission (www.jointcommission.org), which lists hospitals that have certification for various medical specialties; and Hospital Compare (www.hhs

.gov), which gives detailed information about procedures performed at different hospitals.

If the information you're looking for isn't available on the Internet, you can call the hospital's quality office. Dr. Collier says you should ask about volume; studies show that hospitals that perform a high number of a given procedure—say, heart-bypass or hip-replacement surgery—usually have the best results. The Leapfrog Group and HealthGrades have information about what constitutes high volume for various procedures, and they also have information about staffing, which plays a key role. "Let's say I'm having a surgery where it's highly likely I'm going to have a stay in the intensive-care unit," said Suzanne Delbanco, a CEO at the Leapfrog Group. "Your risk of dying in an ICU drops forty percent if the doctors working there are 'intensivists,' which means they have specialty training in critical care. Ask if they have that kind of staffing."

GETTING THE CARE YOU NEED IN THE EMERGENCY ROOM

For several "Empowered Patient" columns, I've asked emergency-room physicians for tips on how to avoid long waits in the emergency room. They had all sorts of suggestions that would never have occurred to me, and some of them are quite simple. For example, while you're on your way to the hospital, call your family doctor and ask him to call the ER; ER doctors tell me that when they hear from a fellow physician, they listen. "They'll talk to me professionally and put a bug in my ear," says ER physician David Beiser. "This guy will now be on my radar screen." Here's another thing to do (or not to do) when you're en route to the hospital: don't use an ambulance unless you really need it. "There's a myth out there that if you arrive in an ambulance you'll go straight back to the doctor," says Donna Mason, a former president of the Emergency Nurses Association. It's not true.

Once you arrive at the ER, here are three pieces of advice you should follow. One, don't be quiet. If you're not getting service, make some noise, advises Dr. Assaad Sayah, who runs three emergency rooms for the Cambridge Health Alliance in Massachusetts. "Speak up. Say, 'I need to see the person in charge,' " he says. If the condition of the person you brought in has become worse, say so. Two, don't get angry, and don't lie. While you're making yourself heard, observe the principles of basic human etiquette. "We're all human, and usually when people are nice to us we're nicer to them," Dr. Sayah says. Number three, don't forget the hospital's house phone. If things get really bad and no one is helping you, look for a house phone, dial zero, and ask for the hospital administrator on call. "Even the smallest hospitals have a hospital administrator or a patient advocate on call 24/7," Dr. Sayah says. "Hospital administrators don't want to hear that patients are unhappy. Their job is to break through the hurdles and move forward."

MAKING SURE YOU GET THE RIGHT MEDICINE IN THE HOSPITAL

Avoiding a hospital medication error starts with one basic step: make sure the medicine you've been given is really yours. In chapter 1, we saw how Evan Handler received a drug that wasn't meant for him, and Hedy Cohen, a vice president of the Institute for Safe Medication Practices, witnessed the same thing when she was a hospital nurse. "I personally saw a mom say to a nurse, 'Hey, the IV bag you're about to give my son has another child's name on it,' " she recalls. You should also ask your doctor or nurse every day for a schedule of the medications you're supposed to receive, along with the dosage and what the medicine looks like. "That way, if you're supposed to get an orange pill at noon and instead you get a blue one, you can say something," Cohen says.

The next step is to check off whenever a dose of a medicine is given so that it won't be given again. Dr. Albert Wu, a professor at the Johns Hopkins School of Public Health, says that he kept track of medications when his wife, Diana Sugg, was in the hospital and prevented a nurse from giving her a double dose; the nurse was about to give her antibiotics intravenously when she had just taken the same antibiotic in pill form. "Had I not been there to intercept the error, she would have gotten both doses," he says.

If you think you're getting the wrong medicine (or at the wrong time or the wrong dosage) and the nurse won't listen to you, get dramatic if you have to. Dr. Wu says when the young daughter of a friend of his was in the hospital his friend realized that a nurse was about to give his daughter the wrong medicine. When Wu's friend told the nurse this was not the medication the doctor had ordered, she didn't believe him. "He threw himself across the bed until they realized the medication was for the next patient," Wu says. Hopefully you won't have to use your body to stop a nurse from doing the wrong thing. "You could say, 'Just to be safe, could you please check with the doctor,' " Wu advises. "Say, 'I don't want anything bad to happen, so please check.' "

MAKING SURE YOU'RE NOT CONFUSED
WITH ANOTHER PATIENT IN THE HOSPITAL

When Kerry Higuera started bleeding three months into her pregnancy, she feared she was miscarrying. When she arrived at the ER, she was put in a room and told to wait for a nurse to come for her. Soon, a nurse poked her head into the room. "She said, 'Kerry?' and I said, 'Yes.' She said, 'I'm going to take you for a little walk,' and I followed her down the hallway," Kerry recalls. "She brought me to the CT-scan room, and I said, 'Is this really what I need to have done?' And the nurse said, 'Yes, this is what the doctor wants. He wants a CT scan of your abdomen,' and I said, 'Okay.' "

After the scan, the nurse led Kerry back to a room to wait for the doctor, and Kerry and her husband were sure they were about to hear that the CT scan showed they'd lost the baby. But that's not what happened. After about half an hour of waiting, Kerry says the emergency-room physician, two radiologists, and a representative from the hospital's human-resources department came into her room. "I started to cry and asked if I'd miscarried, and they said no, I was still pregnant. My husband and I said, 'Oh, that's great!' " she recalls. But then they told the Higueras there was something else they needed to know. "They said, 'We made a mistake; we did something we shouldn't have done.' I was, like, 'What do you mean?' " Kerry says. "They said, 'There's another patient here named Kerry, and you two are the same age. We mixed you up. She was supposed to have the CT scan, not you.' " I got a look at Kerry's hospital records, and one doctor's note says it all: "The patient was unintentionally scanned, as she was confused with another patient." Fifteen months later, Higuera's son, Nathan, is showing signs of developmental delays, and she's considering a lawsuit against the hospital.

Kerry's situation is far more common than you might think. More than five times a day, wrong-patient, wrong-side, or wrong-site procedures occur in U.S. hospitals, according to the Joint Commission. Sometimes a right knee is operated on instead of a left knee; at other times a patient goes in for eye surgery and gets his tonsils out instead. (I'm not making this up—it actually happened at a hospital in Rhode Island.)

There are several steps you can take to ensure that you and your family don't receive the wrong surgery. First, say, "My name is Mary Smith, my date of birth is October 21, 1965, and I'm here for an appendectomy" to every doctor, nurse, and technician who comes to take care of you. You'll feel like an idiot, but you won't be mistaken for someone else. (And, come to think of it, if your name really is Mary Smith, you might want to add your middle initial!) Also, ask hospital staff to check your ID bracelet before they do anything to you, whether it's giving you a drug or sending you for a CT scan. If you're having surgery, your hospital might give you a pen and ask you to mark the site where the surgery is supposed to be performed. That's a great idea, but make sure you make the mark in the presence of the surgeon. Marking the site in front of a pre-op nurse isn't enough, because she may not be in the operating room when the surgery takes place. You want the person who's actually wielding the knife to know what body part he's aiming for.

Finally, it's crucial that you follow your instincts—and be impolite if necessary. Kerry says she wondered why she was having a CT scan when she was pregnant, but acquiesced when the nurse said the doctor had ordered the scan. "If that happened to me now, I would say, 'Stop everything. I'm not doing this scan,'" she told me. "If I was wrong, I'd have been embarrassed. But I'd rather be embarrassed than be in the situation we're in now."

AVOIDING HOSPITAL INFECTIONS

Like many young men, Josh Nahum loved a thrill. But on Labor Day weekend in 2006 Josh had an accident while skydiving in Colorado, fracturing his femur and his skull; he spent six weeks in the intensive-care unit. Slowly, his condition improved, and his doctors predicted a full recovery. But suddenly Josh developed a bacterial infection. He died two weeks later, at the age of twenty-seven. Because of the timing, there's no question that Josh became infected while he was in the hospital. He couldn't have brought the infection with him from outside.

Josh's parents were grief-stricken and horrified when they learned that Josh's death could have been prevented. "One nurse, who was trying to be comforting, said, 'These things happen,'" Victoria Nahum, Josh's stepmother recalls. "That's true, but they happen way more often than they need to happen." After Josh died, the Nahums started the Safe Care Campaign, to get hospitals to do a better job of controlling infections, and also to advise patients about what they can do to avoid becoming victims. Here's what you can do: First, the week before your procedure, ask your surgeon whether you should wash your skin daily with a disinfectant such as chlorhexidine in preparation. Also, ask whether you should have a nasal or skin swab for MRSA, the superbug that causes many hospital infections. If you have MRSA, you can be treated with antibiotics.

Then, the day of surgery—and this sounds strange—heat up your car while you're driving to the hospital. Studies show that staying warm before and during surgery can help you fight infection. The Institute for Healthcare Improvement suggests that in cold weather you heat up the car, wear warm clothes on the way to the hospital, ask the hospital staff to give you plenty of blankets while you wait for surgery, and ask how you'll be kept warm during surgery. When you're being prepared for surgery, if the surgical site needs to be shaved, ask to be clippered, not shaved with a razor, as razors can create nicks where bacteria thrive. Also, on the day of the procedure, if your doctor has ordered IV antibiotics to be administered just before surgery, make sure you get your presurgical antibiotics, as they're sometimes forgotten.

Catheters deserve a special note. A catheter is a thin flexible tube that's inserted into the body, and it can become a breeding ground for bacteria. If you or a loved one has a urinary catheter in the hospital, be vigilant. First, ask if a urinary catheter is truly necessary. "If the patient is awake and oriented and alert and can use a bedpan, it may not be needed," says Dr. John Jernigan, a medical epidemiologist at the Centers for Disease Control and Prevention. If you get one, make sure it comes out ASAP, since the longer it's in, the riskier it becomes. Central venous catheters (also called central lines) can also become breeding grounds for bacteria and cause dangerous bloodstream infections. A central line is inserted into a large vein leading to the heart and used to deliver medications, fluid, or blood. According to the CDC, about 250,000 people get central line–associated bloodstream infections each year, and an estimated 30,000 to 62,000 infected patients die. If the hospital wants to give you a central line, ask if it's necessary, and, if it is, ask how quickly it can be removed. "My brother was in the hospital and needed a central venous catheter for his procedure," Dr. Jernigan recalls. "The day after surgery, I asked the nurse, 'Are you all still using this? Do you still need it?' And she checked and came back and said, 'We don't need it anymore. We'll take it out.' "

You'll stay safer in the hospital if all the people who touch you wash their hands to decrease the chances that you'll get an infection. Hospital workers (doctors, nurses, aids, technicians) should know to wash their hands before touching you, but as we saw from the CDC statistics, many of them don't, so you need to ask hospital workers to wash their hands before they touch you. Victoria Nahum suggests putting your request like this: "I didn't see you wash your hands. Do you mind doing it in front of me?" Many patients (myself included) feel uncomfortable with this direct approach, so I asked Dr. Vicki Rackner, a surgeon and patient advocate, for a few ideas on lightening things up. "In the hospital, you can have the grandkids make a sign that says, 'Please wash your hands and keep Grandma healthy.' " Another suggestion: put a dish of wrapped candy near the sink and say, 'Could you please wash your hands. Oh, and please take some of the candy over there with you when we're done.' "

If the doctor or nurse has gloves on, don't be fooled into thinking gloves make everything okay. When you put gloves on with dirty hands, guess what happens? Right—you get dirty gloves! Last year, when I had to have some chunks of wood removed from the inside of my foot, the podiatrist's assistant walked into the room with gloved hands and started to touch my foot. "Sir, would you mind washing your hands before working on my foot?" I asked politely. He actually argued with me. "I put those gloves on just before I entered your room. They're clean," he said. I asked him again to wash his hands. He stormed out of the room and never returned. Although I felt uncomfortable that he was so upset, at least I got what I wanted: he didn't touch my infected foot with his potentially germy gloves.

After the assistant left, the podiatrist himself came into my room with bare hands, took a pair of gloves from a box on the table, and put it on without washing his hands first. I asked him to take the gloves off, wash his hands, and put on a fresh pair of gloves. He gave me a condescending smirk, but he did as I asked. While I didn't appreciate the attitude, once again I got what I wanted.

Washing Hands: The Howie Mandel Solution

While I was in the hospital with my husband after he had surgery, something happened that bowled me over: doctors and nurses were coming in to check his incision without washing their hands first! I asked them to wash their hands, but I felt uncomfortable doing it.

Then, straight out of the television in my husband's hospital room, Howie Mandel gave me a solution to my problem. Just as yet another nurse was going to touch my husband's incision without first washing her hands, Mandel's game show popped up on the screen. An idea came into my mind. I said to the nurse, "Excuse me, I'm so sorry, but you've heard of Howie Mandel, that crazy germaphobe? Well, I'm like him. I'm totally neurotic about germs. I'm sure your hands are completely clean, but would you mind washing them so I can see? I know it's nuts, but it would make me feel much better." She immediately said, "Oh, of course! No problem!" and washed her hands.

Thank you, Howie, for giving me this great approach!

CONCLUSION: HOSPITALS CAN BE SCARY PLACES

After giving birth to my second daughter, my hand, which had an IV line in it, started to swell up. At first it wasn't a big deal, but over the course of several hours my hand began to really hurt, and it soon looked like a balloon.

I pointed out my swollen, painful hand to the nurse, and she shrugged it off, saying it was normal for a hand with an IV in it to look that way. Finally, when it got to the point that I was in serious pain and I couldn't even lift my hand, I asked the nurse to change the IV, and she said no, that it wasn't necessary. Then I asked her to call in someone from the IV team. (I knew from my hospital stay with my first daughter that there were specialized teams to help with IV lines.) She again said no. I insisted. Finally, she grudgingly agreed. When the IV specialist appeared, he took one look at my hand and said, "That's not supposed to be like that!" He took out the IV and put in a new one. Almost instantly, the swelling subsided and within minutes my hand felt fine.

So why hadn't the nurse changed the IV line the first time I asked her? I think it's because hospitals and the people who work in them have their own systems, their own way of doing things, their own customs, and they're not going to change them for you; after all, this is their world, and you're just visiting it. If a nurse has been putting on gloves without washing her hands for twenty years, she's not going to change now. If a pharmacy technician has stored a bottle of medicine without first taking a close look at the label many times before, he's not likely to start looking now. It takes huge forces to change the little things people have done day in and day out for years, but it's worth making an effort to get them to change. With a little charm and basic human kindness, you'll get your way—and you might save your own life.

Final Checklist: How to Keep a Hospital from Killing You

1. **Choose your hospital wisely.** Not all hospitals are the same: the right hospital can save you, and the wrong hospital can kill you. Some hospitals, for example, are better equipped than others to take care of premature babies or to give the right medicine to someone who has just had a stroke or to put a stent into a patient's heart. To find the hospital that's right for you, check out *U.S. News & World Report*'s top 50 hospitals and visit www .healthgrades.com or www.leapfroggroup.org.

2. **Ask for a daily medication list.** Every morning, ask for a list of medications you'll receive that day, along with the dosages, the time you'll be receiving them, and, if they're not intravenous, what they look like. Then, every time you're given a medicine, make sure this is the drug you're supposed to receive and that you're getting the right dosage. Also, don't forget to check the name on the label—make sure it's yours.

3. **On your way to the emergency room, call your family doctor.** Your family doctor can call ahead so the ER staff knows you're on your way and why you're coming in. On your way to the ER, don't use an ambulance unless you really need to (you'll just make the staff mad).

4. **Don't be quiet in the emergency room.** If you're not seen in a timely manner, speak up. Ask to talk to the person in charge, but don't get angry and don't say that you have symptoms you don't really have just to make your situation sound more urgent than it is. If the person you brought in is getting worse, say so. If you don't get a response, look for a house phone, dial zero, and ask for the hospital administrator on call.

5. **A week before surgery, ask your doctor these questions.** The week before your procedure is scheduled, ask your surgeon whether you should wash your skin daily with a disinfectant like

chlorhexidine to prevent infections. Also, ask whether you should have a nasal or skin swab for MRSA, the superbug that causes many hospital infections.

6. **In the hospital, do what you can to prevent infections.** If necessary, before surgery, ask to be clippered, not shaved with a razor, as razors can create nicks where bacteria thrive. Also, if you're told that you need a urinary catheter, ask if it's truly necessary, since catheters can become sites of infection. If you need a catheter, make sure it comes out as soon as possible.

7. **Ask the people who touch you to wash their hands first.** Don't let a doctor, nurse, technician, or anyone else touch you unless you've seen them wash or sanitize their hands. If someone walks in with gloves and wants to touch you, that's not good enough. If someone walks into your room with bare hands and puts on a pair of gloves, that's not good enough, either. If those hands are dirty, they've now soiled the gloves. The bottom line: you want to personally see hospital staff members wash or sanitize their hands every time they touch you.

Epilogue

Looking back, I can see now that this book was born on Friday, August 22, 1997, at 2 P.M. with a loud rip of Velcro. Hot, sweaty, and nearly eight weeks away from my due date with my first child, I sat in my obstetrician's office as the nurse tore off the blood-pressure cuff she'd just wrapped around my arm. "This reading can't be right," she said. "You're a little person—I must need a smaller cuff." She found one, but the result was the same: 150/90 when at all my previous visits my blood pressure had been more like 100/60. She asked me how I'd been feeling. I told her not great—tired and sluggish, but it was Atlanta, it was August, and I was eight months' pregnant. The nurse disappeared, and as I looked around the corner I could see her conferring with the obstetrician, who came back to take my blood pressure himself. The reading didn't change. "You have preeclampsia," he told me.

Preeclampsia is a serious disease of pregnancy. In addition to the elevated blood pressure, I had high levels of protein in my urine whereas in a normal pregnancy a woman has none, or nearly none. "You may have the baby this weekend," my doctor told me as he picked up the phone to tell the hospital I was on my way. I was confused. "It's August, and I'm not due until October. How could I have the baby now?" I asked. He explained to me that the only way to make the preeclampsia go away was to deliver the baby. And at a certain point, you have to make preeclampsia go away. If the disease goes unchecked, both the mother and the baby can die.

So after a week's stay in the hospital, when my blood pressure and protein levels climbed out of control, the doctors performed a Cesarean section, and Tav Rachel Cohen was born seven weeks early, weighing three pounds even. The doctors had told us that because she was so little and so early we shouldn't expect to hear her cry. Tav apparently wasn't listening, though, and immediately after birth she let out a mighty wail. "Is that our baby?" I asked. "Yes, that's your baby," the doctors and nurses answered. "Are you sure it's not the baby crying in the next room?" I asked. "Yes, we're sure." Tav's cry was the sweetest sound my husband and I had ever heard.

After her birth, Tav went to the neonatal intensive-care unit, and I was sent back to the high-risk-pregnancy floor to recover. Moms with preeclampsia usually get better after giving birth, but instead of getting better, I got worse. I became extremely weak, too weak even to sit up and take a sip of water, and I couldn't keep my eyes open. I wasn't sleepy—I just somehow couldn't muster the strength to keep them open.

Tav was born the Thursday night before Labor Day weekend, and our own obstetrician, who had done such a thoughtful, thorough job of catching the preeclampsia and delivering Tav, went away for the holiday after her delivery. On that Sunday of Labor Day weekend, his colleague who was on call came to my hospital room to see how I was doing. We told him about my weakness, and he nailed the cause immediately. It was a reaction to magnesium sulfate, the medicine that women with preeclampsia are given to prevent seizures. "Mag," as it's called, is a lifesaving medicine, but it can also cause the weakness I was experiencing. I couldn't come off the mag since I might have seizures, but I could get an IV of calcium, which acts as an antidote. The doctor said he'd order a blood test immediately to see if I needed calcium and, if so, how much.

This sounded pretty straightforward: I'd get a blood test, and if it showed that the doctor's hunch was right, I'd get some calcium. At around 11 A.M. the doctor left our room, and we waited for the technician to arrive and draw my blood. We waited. And we waited. Then we waited some more. As the hours passed, I became weaker. In addition to having trouble keeping my eyes open, I couldn't move my arms. Then I couldn't move my legs. Then I became confused about where I was. Meanwhile, tests measuring my liver and kidney function were showing serious damage. The nurses became visibly panicked. "I can't handle taking care of you anymore," one young nurse whispered to me. "I'm handing you over to the head nurse." The head nurse paged the on-call doctor again and again as my condition worsened. My husband, Tal, who was heroically running back and forth between his preemie daughter in intensive care and his rapidly deteriorating wife on the maternity floor, called the doctor's answering service as evening turned to night.

Finally, at around 11 P.M.—twelve hours after the doctor said he'd order the blood test—Tal did the only thing he could think of: he went to the nurse's station and quietly, politely went berserk. He explained that he knew it wasn't the nurses' fault but a doctor hadn't seen me in a long time and they needed to get one into my room, and fast. My mother, who was in the hospital room with us, watched as Tal made his impassioned plea, looking the nurses directly in the eye, agitated but not so crazy that they could write him off as an overly emotional new father. It worked. Within minutes of Tal's plea an obstetrician who specialized in high-risk patients walked through my door. She took one look at me, ordered a calcium test, and a technician arrived within minutes to take my blood. The results arrived quickly: not only was my calcium level low; it was by far the lowest this high-risk doctor had ever seen in a patient in her entire career. She had to give me five times more calcium than she'd ever given anyone else. Within an hour of receiving the calcium, I moved my arms. I moved my legs. I opened my eyes. No one ever explained why it took more than twelve hours to get the medicine I needed.

Two years after Tav's birth, I went back to the same hospital to deliver her little sister, Neri. From my hospital bed, I noticed two nurses pointing at me and whispering. One of them came over to me and said, "We know who you are. You're the one who was so sick a few years ago." It's a bad sign when, in one of the busiest maternity hospitals in the country, the nurses remember you two years later. Ten years after that, I told the story of Tav's birth at a fundraiser for the Preeclampsia Foundation. After my speech, a prominent preeclampsia researcher came up to the podium and shook my hand. "Your doctor was a dumb f——," he said. "And I can't believe you didn't die." It was a strange greeting, but the doctor explained to me that magnesium sulfate, the drug I had been taking, can start to deplete the body of calcium, and your muscles can't function without calcium. Your heart is a muscle like any other. I was extremely lucky, he said, that along with my legs, my arms, and my eyes, my heart didn't stop working. Tal will forever be my hero; if he hadn't had his polite but relentless fit, I might not have received that calcium until it was much too late.

On Tuesday, the day after Labor Day, my regular doctor came back to work and entered our room looking grim. We hadn't spoken to him about the weekend's events, but apparently he'd heard. "I'm so sorry, I'm so sorry, I'm so sorry, I'm so sorry," he said over and over. While we were grateful for the apology, we wondered why it came from a doctor who had nothing to be sorry for—who had in fact done a great job—and why the doctor who was responsible for the potentially deadly twelve-hour calcium delay never expressed a single word of remorse or regret.

As I remember that rip of Velcro, that single sound that started the journey of writing this book, I think about all the people I've met along the way who, like Tal and me, had to force the medical system to do the right thing. I think of Stephanie, the young woman who was six feet tall and weighed 113 pounds because her doctor, for more than ten years, missed the signs of a rather obvious diagnosis. I think of my mother, who might not need a kidney transplant now if her doctor had taken her high blood pressure seriously. I think of Marian Sandmaier, who had to diagnose her daughter's potentially debilitating disease by herself on the Internet, and who got pushback from doctors when she did so. I think of Trisha Torrey, who figured out on her own that she didn't really have cancer when her doctor said she did. I think of Kimberly and Dennis Quaid, watching helplessly as their newborn babies nearly bled to death from a medical mistake.

These journeys, theirs and mine, have led me to four conclusions. Conclusion number one: you should always have someone with you in a medical setting to ask the questions you might not think of and to advocate on your behalf if necessary. Conclusion number two: trust your instincts, because they're almost always right. Conclusion number three: don't be scared to make a fuss when you need to, and keep making that fuss even when you get pushback.

Conclusion number four: listen to Dr. Seuss. This comes to me via Gilles Frydman, the Internet pioneer who started one of the most successful medical websites ever, the Association of Cancer Online Resources. The other day, Gilles pointed out to me that folks like Barbara, Marian, Trisha, the Quaids, and Tal and me each had an "aha!" moment, a specific point in time when something went wrong with our health care and we realized that we needed to become empowered patients. Gilles quoted Dr. Seuss to explain that we're perfectly equipped to take charge, even if we don't always feel that way. In his book *Oh, the Places You'll Go!* the good doctor wrote, "You have brains in your head, you have feet in your shoes, you can steer yourself in any direction you choose. You're on your own. And you know what you know. You are the guy who'll decide where to go."

May you proceed through life in good health, but when you do hit an unhealthy bump in the road, be the guy or gal who decides where to go and what to do. It's your body. It's your health. Doctors and nurses have saved my life and the lives of my daughters, and I'll be forever grateful to them, but sometimes *you* will be the one to save your own life, or the life of someone you love.

Acknowledgments

For nearly twenty years, I've had the honor of working for the finest news organization in the world. I want to thank Jim Walton, president of CNN Worldwide, not only for making our network the most rewarding place in the world to practice journalism but also for fostering a sense of community and affection among the people who work there.

Jon Klein, president of CNN/United States, is the father of *The Empowered Patient,* having encouraged me to start the CNN.com column in 2007. His keen sense of storytelling and high journalist standards have been my guiding light. Many thanks also to Scot Safon, CNN's marketing officer, for his vision and devotion to this project, and to Roni Selig, senior executive producer of CNN's health team, for her energy, leadership, creativity, and friendship. I'm also grateful to Polyanna Dunn and her team at CNN, whose work was indispensible on this project.

I've been blessed with many friends and advisers at CNN, including Rick Davis, Dr. Sanjay Gupta, Nancy Lane, Jay Kernis, Marylynn Ryan, Richard Griffiths, Suzanne Simons, Jeffery Reid, Jennifer Hyde, Michael Schulder, Tim Langmaid, Miriam Falco, and the entire CNN medical team, especially the talented Sabriya Rice and John Bonifield, who work tirelessly for our pieces on television and online. At cnnhealth.com, many thanks to senior producer Mary Carter for being an eagle-eyed, inspirational editor and an enthusiastic early supporter of the Empowered Patient concept, and to Mary and Andrea Kane for their fine editing every Wednesday afternoon.

Many thanks also to my teachers, including John Schuler, Paula Titon, Phyllis Scattergood, and David Rothman, director of the Center for the Study of Society and Medicine at Columbia. Art Caplan, at the University of Pennsylvania, was never officially my teacher, but for more than twenty years he's been my astute guide through the world of medical ethics. George Annas, my adviser while I was at the Boston University School of Public Health, is the nation's beacon on patients' rights issues, and he's been my beacon and inspiration as well. Also thanks to Joseph Harzbecker, the head of reference at Boston University Medical Center, for graciously supplying me with many of the studies cited in this book.

A journalist, I've always known, owes everything to her sources. Over the years, countless people have allowed me into their lives to tell their stories, and I'm grateful to every one of them. A special thanks from the bottom of my heart to Marci and Tim Smith and Jeannie and Nasir Moloo, who spent many hours sharing their experiences and insights with me as they've handled their own medical challenges. Their strength, dignity, energy, and love continue to inspire me. Thanks also to Susannah Fox, Gilles Frydman, Trisha Torrey, "epatient Dave" deBronkart, and other leaders of the empowered-patient movement for sharing their insights with me. Finally, a source from within, Alisha Penick, director of benefits at Turner Broadcasting, has been a huge help in explaining the byzantine system of insurance, including my own.

A journalist, I found out this year, knows very little about writing a book. My literary agent, Lynn Johnston, gave me a quick and thorough education, answering calls at all hours and speaking with great intelligence and insight even when she was competing with four loud juvenile voices in the background on my side of the conversation. Thank you, Lynn, for your dedication and your keen eye, your encouragement and your conviction that I could help people with this book.

When Lynn set me up with Jill Schwartzman at Random House, I knew right away that I'd landed with the right editor. Thank you, Jill, for your tireless hard work ushering me through this process and shaping my prose into an actual book. I couldn't have asked for a better editor.

Liza Hogan, a dear friend and a sharp-eyed wordsmith, tore herself away from her own work and children to read large portions of my manuscript. Thank you, Liza, for your suggestions, all of which were right on the mark. Two other wonderful friends, Jodi Fleisig and Greg McCarthy, also provided invaluable advice and were generous with their time. I'm grateful also to John Bonifield, who copyedited the chapter on prescription drugs and was kind enough not to charge me twenty dollars as he did in college when he read his friends' term papers. Many thanks to Connie Glaser and David Munn, who gave me strategic advice and cheerleading in abundance, and to Jolene Eyre Postley, who has style in spades in every way.

Many thanks to my siblings, Pamela and Steve Cohen, Jane Price and David Schwartz, Julia and John Healy, Alumit and Oded Gour-Lavie, and to Ofra and Guy Tessler, and Nissim Harel, who technically aren't my siblings but might as well be. I'm grateful to my cousin David Kanter for giving me much-needed computer guidance, and to another cousin, Ron Ansin, for his advice and inspiration, and to my mother-in-law, Yaffa Cohen, for her love, wisdom, good cooking, and devotion to our family. Words cannot express my gratitude to my parents, Sheila and Charles Schwartz. Their loving support of their children has meant everything, and those dinner-table discussions about medical and legal ethics as we were growing up really did amount to something!

Our four daughters, Tav, Neri, Shir, and Yaara, have been jumping-up-and-down excited about this book, even when it meant that I had to spend time away from them with my nose in my computer. Thank you, girls. You're the best, and the light of our lives.

A few months ago, one of my daughters made a wise suggestion: "Mom, if you don't dedicate the book to us you should dedicate it to Jen." Jennifer Bixler, executive producer at CNN Medical, has been the best colleague anyone could ever ask for. The other mother to the "Empowered Patient" column, she's shaped and nurtured the concept from the beginning. I won the professional lottery the day we began working together.

I won the life lottery on an unseasonably warm day in December 1991, when I met my husband, Tal, at a random holiday party. This book truly wouldn't exist without him. He suggested that I write it and pushed me when I thought I couldn't; he read the manuscript several times and changed its course; and he took our children to every conceivable fair, festival, and museum in the state of Georgia so I could write it. He also saved my life, so I dedicate this book, and my heart, to him.

Appendix

WEBSITES FOR CHECKING OUT YOUR DOCTOR

These are all free websites. Since these sites are pretty big, I've told you what to Google in order to get to the exact page.

1. **Federation of State Medical Boards (www.fsmb.org)** Go here to find out if there have been any disciplinary actions against a doctor. Google "Federation of State Medical Boards directory" and you'll get an alphabetical list of state medical boards.

2. **American Board of Medical Specialties (www.abms.org)** All doctors have to be licensed to practice medicine by a state medical board. Some, in addition, choose to go a step further and receive board certification in their particular specialty (pediatrics, obstetrics and gynecology, internal medicine, etc.). You don't absolutely have to have a doctor who's board certified, but this ensures that he has had specialized training and has taken certain exams in his field. Google "ABMS is your doctor certified" and that'll take you directly to the right page. You'll have to create a login and a password, but access to the site is free, quick, and easy.

3. **Office of the Inspector General (www.oig.hhs.gov)** The Office of the Inspector General, a part of the federal Depart-

ment of Health and Human Services, keeps a list of doctors who have been kicked out of the federal Medicaid or Medicare program because they've been convicted of fraud or patient abuse or have defaulted on their loans. If the feds don't want to use them, you might not want to, either. Google "OIG HHS exclusion searchable database" and you'll go right to the page where you can put in a doctor's name to see if she's on the list.

"GET IT DUN!" WORKSHEET

When you're in the examining room, make sure you get your business DUN: find out your **diagnosis, understand** the plan to make you better, and learn the **next steps** toward making you feel better. This worksheet is bare-bones, because when you're in the doctor's office, with just minutes to understand what she's saying, you want something very clean and easy to consult. If you've got more time, or a more complicated situation, by all means ask more questions. You can print out more of these worksheets at my website: www.elizabethcohen.com.

D—Diagnosis
1. What's my diagnosis?

_____

_____

U–Understand the Plan to Get Me Better
1. Which drugs should I take, if any?

_____

_____

2. Are there any other treatments or instructions?

_____

_____

3. Do I need a specialist? If so, do you have a specific recommendation?

_____

_____

N—Next Steps

1. How long should I wait for this treatment to work?

_____

_____

2. If my problem doesn't get better in that time, what should I do?

_____

_____

3. Am I awaiting any test results? If so, when are they due back in your office?

_____

_____

A SAMPLE "GET IT DUN!" CONVERSATION AND WORKSHEET

MRS. MOM has brought her baby in to see the pediatrician because the baby is unusually fussy and keeps tugging on her ears. She's a "Get It DUN!" mom, so she has brought in a blank "Get It DUN!" worksheet, and after the conversation you'll see how she fills it out. Remember, D stands for diagnosis, U for understand the plan to get you better, and N for next steps.

DR. DOCTOR: Mrs. Mom, your baby needs to take this antibiotic for an ear infection (handing over prescription). Here you go. See you later.

MRS. MOM: Thank you, Doctor. I have a few questions. So she has an ear infection. Anything else, or is that it?

DR. DOCTOR: She may have a urinary-tract infection.

MRS. MOM: Okay, so she has an ear infection and possibly a urinary-tract infection. (Get it DUN—there's the *D*!) You're prescribing an antibiotic—should that take care of both problems?

DR. DOCTOR: Yes, that should do it. (Get it DUN—there's the *U*! Now Mrs. Mom understands the plan to get her baby better.)

MRS. MOM: Okay, so when I leave here I'm going to get the prescription filled. How will I know if it's working?

DR. DOCTOR: She should feel better in the next forty-eight hours or so.

MRS. MOM: And if she's not?

DR. DOCTOR: Call me. She might need a different antibiotic.

MRS. MOM: Okay. And what are the next steps regarding the possible urinary-tract infection?

DR. DOCTOR: I took some urine from her today to find out if she has an infection. I should have the results back in two days. We'll call you, and if she does have one, I may need to prescribe a different antibiotic.

MRS. MOM: Okay, so the immediate plan is she's taking antibiotics, I should call you in two days if she's not feeling better, and you'll be calling me at that time anyway to tell me about the urine-test results. (Get it DUN—there's the *N*!)

DR. DOCTOR: That's right.

MOM: Anything else?

DR. DOCTOR: Yes, I think you should put a humidifier in her room.

MRS. MOM: Great. Thanks, Doctor.

MRS. MOM'S FILLED-IN "GET IT DUN!" WORKSHEET

D—Diagnosis

1. What's my diagnosis?
   Ear infection.

U—Understand the Plan to Get Me Better

1. What drugs should I take, if any?

   <u>Amoxicillin, six milliliters every morning and evening for ten days.</u>

2. Are there any other treatments or instructions?

   <u>Use a humidifier in the room so she can breathe more easily.</u>

3. Do I need a specialist? If so, do you have a specific recommendation?

   <u>No.</u>

N—Next Steps

1. How long should I wait for this treatment to work?

   <u>Two days.</u>

2. If my problem doesn't get better in that time, what should I do?

   <u>Call the doctor—I might need a new antibiotic.</u>

3. Am I awaiting any test results? If so, when are they due back in your office?

   <u>The test for urinary-tract infection is due back on Wednesday. Call the doctor at the end of the day on Wednesday if he hasn't called me.</u>

SPECIAL QUESTIONS FOR COMPLICATED PROBLEMS

With a complicated problem, you'll have more success at the doctor's office if you come prepared. Here's a list of questions to ask yourself before your appointment.

1. What are my symptoms?

   _____

   _____

2. When did they begin?

   _____

   _____

3. What brings on the symptoms?

   _____

   _____

4. What diagnoses have other doctors given me?

   _____

   _____

5. In the past, what helped to relieve my symptoms?

   _____

   _____

6. What didn't help to relieve or get rid of my symptoms?

   _____

   _____

   Questions to ask yourself before a follow-up visit:

7. The treatment recommended at the last visit—has it worked?

   _____

   _____

8. Has the treatment been causing me any problems?

   _____

   _____

9. Have I noticed any new symptoms since my last visit?

   _____

   _____

10. Have I heard of any new treatments that I want to ask my doctor about?

    _____

    _____

A SAMPLE CONVERSATION ABOUT MONEY
WITH YOUR DOCTOR

DOCTOR: Here's a prescription for an antidepressant. Come back in two weeks and tell me how it's going.

YOU: Doctor, I feel really uncomfortable talking about this, but we all need to save money. Here's a list of $4 generics at my pharmacy. Do you mind if we take a minute and see if the drug you're prescribing is on this list?

DOCTOR (*taking the list*): Sure. Hmm . . . it's not on there.

YOU: I'm worried, because I don't have great prescription-drug insurance. I'm not sure I can afford the drug you're prescribing for me. Do you see one on that list that would work for me?

DOCTOR: No. I think the drug I've prescribed is the best antidepressant for you.

YOU: I really appreciate that you're trying to give me the best drug. But I'm wondering, I've never tried an antidepressant before, and might there be one that works as well as the one you want me to take? Is there another reasonable choice? The price difference could be huge.

DOCTOR: Well, maybe there is. But I don't know what your insurance will pay for and won't pay for.

YOU: I understand. Before I came here I called my insurance company, since I knew I might need an antidepressant. Here's a list of the company's three cheapest antidepressants. I hate to make money such an issue, but I know that I might need this drug for months or even years, and I want to be able to afford to keep taking it.

DOCTOR: Okay, this one might work for you. Here's a prescription for it. But remember, please come back and tell me how you're doing on it. We might still have to switch you to the more expensive one.

HOW TO GET OUT OF MEDICAL DEBT

It took the Trim family of Arlington, Texas, exactly three hours to incur $15,000 in medical debt. It happened when Gayle and Calvin Trim's teenage son, Alex, was hit by a car while riding his bike; while Alex was fine, the bill nearly gave Calvin a heart attack when it arrived in the mail. "I didn't have a clue you could get into debt for $15,000 in one night," Calvin told me. "When I saw that bill, I was just kind of numb." This didn't even include bills from the doctors and the ambulance service. The Trims knew they were in trouble: Alex was uninsured. Gayle had just started a job as an executive assistant at a commercial real-estate company and wasn't yet eligible for insurance. The Trims said they couldn't afford to put Alex on the insurance Calvin gets from the school where he works, because they still owed $1,100 from when Calvin had kidney stones a few months earlier.

The Trims are not alone. A 2008 report from the Commonwealth Fund found that more than one in four Americans is paying off medical debt. That year, an estimated 72 million Americans reported that they were struggling to pay their medical bills or had medical debts they couldn't pay. People with medical debt face awful choices. Nearly one-third of those with medical debt were unable to pay for food, rent, or heat, and some even took out a mortgage or a loan against their home in order to pay this debt. Part of the problem is that often insurance companies refuse to pay for legitimate charges, and you get saddled with the bill; nearly one out of every four Americans has had a legitimate claim denied, according to a survey by PNC Financial Services Group.

In fact, having insurance is no guarantee that you won't get into medical debt. "Two-thirds of the people who go into medical debt have insurance," said Mark Rukavina, the executive director of the Access Project, which works to improve access to healthcare. "When medical debt hits, it hits very quickly. It's a jolt, and it's generally not very predictable," Jessie Maurer, a medical billing advocate in Iowa, added. "These are all honest, hardworking people. This could happen to just about anybody."

To get out of medical debt, do what the Trims did and face your bills head-on, instead of stuffing them in a desk drawer. "The most dangerous thing people do when they get into debt is ignore the statements and notices," said Mary Jean Geroulo, a former hospital administrator who's now a partner at Stewart Stimmel, a health-care law firm in Dallas, Texas. "They think doctors and hospitals won't send them to collection agencies, but they absolutely will."

Your next step is to ask for an itemized copy of your bill to check for accuracy. You might be shocked by what you see. "I had a client once who was charged for a surgery she never had," said Nora Johnson, the vice president of Medical Billing Advocates of America in Caldwell, West Virginia. "Another one was charged more than $5,000 for disposable gloves." The Trims hired Jessie Maurer to help them go through their bills, and she caught about $3,000 in errors and was able to get the bill down from $15,000 to $12,000.

Now it's time to negotiate with doctors and hospitals. You'd be surprised how well this can work. "People think they have to pay the amount on the bill. But doctors and hospitals are very willing to negotiate," Mark Rukavina says. "Remember, the squeaky wheel gets the grease." Maurer remembers a client who owed $14,000 for a five-hour stay in a hospital emergency room. "She could afford to pay $4,000, so I told her, 'Show them a certified check for $4,000.' She did, and told them, 'This is all I have in the world,' and they took it." Just by asking, Maurer got the hospital that treated Alex Trim to cut $2,000 off the bill, getting the total down to $10,000. Maurer arranged to have the Trims pay this balance in $250 interest-free monthly installments. For more tips on negotiating, read the book *My Healthcare Is Killing Me*; there's a free version online (www.myhealthcareiskillingme.com).

You can do all this checking and negotiating on your own, or you can find a medical billing advocate to help you. To find one, visit the website of Medical Billing Advocates of America. The Fairness Foundation, the National Foundation for Credit Counseling, and the Patient Advocate Foundation also offer help to those in debt.

THEY SAY, YOU SAY: SAMPLE CONVERSATIONS FOR GETTING WHAT YOU NEED IN THE HOSPITAL

Hospitals can be tough places. Here's what to say when things aren't going well.

1. **They say: "You're having this procedure now" (and you know they're not right).**
   You say: "Check the chart. And check it again."
   When Molly Atryzek was seventeen and entered a Boston hospital to be treated for leukemia, a nurse came into her room to do a bone-marrow extraction, a painful procedure. Her father, Vladimir, knew it wasn't time to do another extraction; he told the nurse Molly had just had one done the day before. The nurse didn't believe him, and insisted on doing the extraction. "I asked the nurse to check [the chart] and she came back and said, 'Oh, you're right. No bone marrow today.' " Oops!

2. **They say: "You don't need pain medication."**
   You say: "Oh, yes I do."
   While she was in the hospital, Molly needed to have a chest tube removed, another painful procedure. Neither the doctor nor the nurse wanted to sedate Molly, even though she'd been sedated for similar procedures before. "I told them eight times, 'No, no, no, she needs to be sedated,' " Suzanne Atryzek, Molly's mother, recalls. Finally, after about thirty minutes of arguing, the doctor and the nurse agreed to sedate Molly.

3. **They say, "Blah-blah-blah, doctor gobbledygook, yada yada yada."**

   You say: "Excuse me? I don't speak doctorese."

   How can you make sure the nurses are doing the right things—giving you the right medications, performing the right procedures—if you don't understand the doctor's orders? When Betty Garrett's husband was in the hospital, a doctor launched into a complicated explanation of his upcoming cancer treatments. "He looked at me and said, 'Do you have any questions?' and I said, 'Yes. What did you just say? I don't have a PhD.'" The doctor then repeated everything in English.

4. **They say something overwhelming and scary.**

   You go to find a smart nurse.

   Late one night, a medical resident came into Molly Atryzek's room and delivered horrible news to her parents: a blood test showed that her cancer was getting worse. Her mother broke down in tears. "But then I went and found a wonderful, smart, smart nurse and got her to explain it to me," Suzanne recalls. The tests didn't actually mean what the resident had said. The next morning, another doctor confirmed that the tests weren't bad news. "Nurses will guide you," says Suzanne, who spent many months in the hospital with Molly. "Nurses are where it's at."

5. **Doctor No. 17 says: "Here's the plan."**

   You say: "Don't tell me. Tell my designated doctor."

   Especially with a long, complicated illness, you're going to have lots of doctors traipsing in and out of your hospital room. Sometimes they give you wrong or contradictory information, as the medical resident did when he misinterpreted Molly's lab results. Do what the Atryzeks did: they picked their favorite doctor and instructed everyone else to talk to her. "I told them, 'Please don't talk to me. Everything goes through Katherine. Please tell her and she'll tell me.' " Katherine could then screen what each doctor said and tell the Atryzeks exactly what they needed to know in terms they could understand.

LONG WAITS IN THE EMERGENCY ROOM: ER DOCTORS TELL YOU WHAT THEY WOULD DO

I asked four ER doctors what they would do if their spouse had a life-threatening emergency and they were facing a long wait in an emergency room. Although all the doctors pointed out that emergency rooms do an excellent job of triaging patients, and you might be waiting because there are more urgent cases ahead of you, they did tell me steps you can take if you truly fear that your loved one isn't getting the care he needs.

Dr. Assaad Sayah, chief of emergency medicine, Cambridge Health Alliance, Massachusetts

"I would start by saying to the triage nurse, 'I know that you are busy, but I need one minute of your time. My wife has been waiting for a long time, and her condition has gotten worse since we arrived.' Describe her worsening condition and say, 'I would really appreciate it if you could take a minute to look at her again.'

"This would work most of the time. If I got a hostile answer, I would ask to speak with the charge nurse or charge physician. If I felt like I was not getting anywhere, I would ask to speak with the administrator on call. The last resort is to call the hospital operator (dial 0 from the phone in the waiting room of the Emergency Department) and ask to have the patient advocate or hospital administrator paged. . . . I would not use inappropriate or threatening language."

Dr. Jesse Pines, assistant professor of emergency medicine, Hospital of the University of Pennsylvania

"A basic principle of medical care is that the squeaky wheel gets the grease. I would recommend advocating on behalf of your spouse. It's uncomfortable that it has to be this way, but it works the same in any service business. The more you complain, the faster the service. But it's a fine line. Complaining can piss off the staff, so it's important not to go over the top. Family members who are too vocal are sometimes escorted out by security. You could say, 'She's not acting right. This is not normal for her.' "

Dr. Joseph Guarisco, chief of emergency services at Ochsner Health System, Louisiana

"I would ask to speak with the Emergency Department director. If they aren't there, I would ask to speak with the charge nurse or shift supervisor. . . . I would advise them that you think the patient has an 'emergency medical condition that should be evaluated right away.' Most of us in emergency medicine define the urgency in those terms and should be responsive.

"If you don't get a response, advise the individual in charge dispassionately and without confrontation: 'I understand you are busy, but I feel the patient will have a bad outcome if she isn't seen right away.' If the person in charge was a nurse, ask to speak with the physician and repeat the same thing. If there's no response, further advise the individual in charge: 'I feel strongly about this and must call the administrator on duty.' If no response, I would call the hospital administrator on call and advise him or her of those same concerns. And mentioning the administrator's name [if you know it] always helps. It should not be necessary. But if you truly feel the patient may suffer harm by not being seen right away, do it."

Dr. David Beiser, assistant professor of medicine,
University of Chicago Medical Center

"If you are concerned that a family member or friend is getting sicker while awaiting treatment in the Emergency Department, it's always reasonable to request that the triage nurse do a quick re-assessment of the patient. Belligerence, histrionics, or requests for VIP treatment usually end up working against the doctor-patient relationship."

Notes

Introduction

xii   **99,000 Americans die each year**   "Estimates of Healthcare-Associated Infections," U.S. Centers for Disease Control and Prevention, June 15, 2009.

xii   **98,000 die from medical mistakes**   Linda Kohn et al., "To Err Is Human: Building a Safer Health System" (Washington, DC: National Academies Press, 2000), 26.

xii   **kill more people**   Cancer Facts & Figures 2009 (Atlanta: American Cancer Society, 2009), 4. "2008 Traffic Safety Annual Assessment—Highlights," National Highway Transportation Safety Administration, June 2009, 1. "HIV/AIDS in the United States," Centers for Disease Control and Prevention, www.cdc.gov. "Leading Causes of Death," Centers for Disease Control and Prevention, www.cdc.gov.

xii   **one out of every four**   Gordon D. Schiff et al., "Diagnosing Diagnosis Errors: Lessons from a Multi-Institutional Collaborative Project," *Advances in Patient Safety: From Research to Implementation,* vol. 2, *Concepts and Methodology,* U.S. Agency for Healthcare Research and Quality, www.ahrq.gov (February 2005): 256.

xii   **one time out of ten**   Stephen S. Raab et al., "Clinical Impact and Frequency of Anatomic Pathology," *Cancer,* 104, no. 10 (November 2005): 2205–13.

xii   **doctor will never call**   Lawrence P. Casalino et al., "Frequency of Failure to Inform Patients of Clinically Significant Outpatient Test Results," *Archives of Internal Medicine* 169, no. 12 (June 2009): 1123–29.

xii   **Women are less likely**   "Women and Heart Disease Facts," Women's Heart Foundation, www.womensheart.org.

xii   **African-Americans are less likely**   Jeff Whittle et al., "Racial Differences in the Use of Invasive Cardiovascular Procedures in the Department of Veterans Affairs Medical System," *New England Journal of Medicine,* 329, no. 9 (August 1993): 621–27.

xiii **spend time with overweight patients** M. R. Hebl and J. Xu, "Weighing the Care: Physicians' Reactions to the Size of a Patient," *International Journal of Obesity* 25, no. 8 (August 2001): 1246–52.

Chapter 1: How to Be a "Bad Patient"

3 **"Doctors told me"** Evan Handler to author, September 19, 2008.

3 **Several times in the hospital** Evan Handler, *Time on Fire: My Comedy of Terrors* (Boston: Little, Brown, 1996), 46–47.

4 **he became exasperated** Handler, *Time on Fire,* 98.

4 **"Nothing bad"** Handler to author, September 19, 2008.

4 **"The irony"** Handler to author.

4 **"I learned that"** Handler, *Time on Fire,* 49–50.

4 **"I was his protector"** Glenn Collins, "How an Actor Found Comedy and Tragedy in Battling Leukemia," *New York Times,* May 12, 1993.

5 **"I barely get to see"** Reader's comment to Elizabeth Cohen, "Are You an Obnoxious Patient?" www.cnn.com/empoweredpatient, January 24, 2008.

5 **"I can't think"** Reader's comment to Cohen, "Are You an Obnoxious Patient?"

5 **"The doctor gave us"** Reader's comment to Cohen, "Five Ways to Find Dr. Right," www.cnn.com/empoweredpatient, February 14, 2008.

5 **doctors who missed their cancer** Reader's comment to Elizabeth Cohen, "Five Symptoms Men Shouldn't Ignore," www.cnn.com/empoweredpatient, June 12, 2008.

5 **pharmacies that gave them** Reader's comment to Elizabeth Cohen, "Is Grandma Drugged Up?" www.cnn.com/empoweredpatient, May 28, 2008.

5 **medical records that were confused** Reader's comment to Cohen, "Are You an Obnoxious Patient?"

5 **surgeons who nearly operated** Reader's comment to Elizabeth Cohen, "Don't Become the Victim of a Surgical Error," www.cnn.com/empoweredpatient, July 17, 2008.

5 **and even a surgeon who performed** Reader's comment to Cohen, "Don't Become the Victim of a Surgical Error."

5 **"Doctors need to get over themselves"** Reader's comment to Cohen, "Are You an Obnoxious Patient?"

5 **"Doctors don't care"** Reader's comment to Cohen, "Five Symptoms Men Shouldn't Ignore."

5–6 **"Doctors think they are gods"** Reader's comment to Elizabeth Cohen, "Five Mistakes Women Make at the Doctor's Office," www.cnn.com/empoweredpatient, May 15, 2008.

6 **"Doctors are generally idiots"** Reader's comment to Elizabeth Cohen, "When It's OK to Question Your Pediatrician's Advice," www.cnn.com/empoweredpatient, March 13, 2008.

6   **"Awww, your malpractice insurance"**   Reader's comment to Cohen, "Are You an Obnoxious Patient?"

7   **Even the president**   *Chicago Sun-Times,* "Obama's AMA Speech as Delivered," June 15, 2009.

7   **when her daughter Stephanie**   Cohen, "Five Mistakes Women Make at the Doctor's Office." Also, Barbara to author, September 11, 2008. Stephanie to author, September 26, 2008.

9   **A 2009 study by doctors**   Lawrence P. Casalino et al., "Frequency of Failure to Inform Patients of Clinically Significant Outpatient Test Results," 1123–29.

10   **a study published**   Brian W. Jack et al., "A Reengineered Hospital Discharge Program to Decrease Rehospitalization," *Annals of Internal Medicine* 150, no. 3 (February 3, 2009): 178–87.

11   **"Disempowerment adds to a patient's distress"**   Elizabeth Cohen, "Empowered Heroes' Lessons Now Help Others," www.cnn.com/empoweredpatient, July 3, 2008.

12   **"Look. You're sick"**   Jerome Groopman to author, August 13, 2007.

12   **"the fog of the examining room"**   Elizabeth Cohen, "Help! I'm Not Feeling Better!" www.cnn.com/empoweredpatient, December 6, 2007.

13   **"You know what"**   Stephanie to author, September 26, 2008.

Chapter 2: How to Find Dr. Right (and Fire Dr. Wrong)

14   **While she's waiting**   Jennifer Crittenden, "The Package," *Seinfeld,* Castle Rock Entertainment, season 8, episode 5 (original aired October 17, 1996).

15   **One day she arrived**   Jennifer Crittenden to author, October 28, 2008.

17   **says she owes her life**   Elizabeth Cohen, "The Life and Death of an Empowered Patient," www.cnn.com/empoweredpatient, February 26, 2009.

19   **"I ask doctors"**   Jennifer Griggs to author, September 3, 2008.

19   **"Turkeys," "trolls," "crocks," and "GOMERS"**   Edward Shahady, "Difficult Patients: Uncovering the Real Problems of 'Crocks' and 'Gomers,' " *Consultant,* October 1990, 49–56. For more on "difficult patients," see Sean Schafer and David P. Nowlis, "Personality Disorders Among Difficult Patients," *Archives of Family Medicine* 7, no. 2 (March/April 1998): 126–29. Leonard J. Haas and Jennifer P. Leiser, "Management of the Difficult Patient," *American Family Physician* 72, no. 10 (November 2005): 2063–68. James E. Groves, "Taking Care of the Hateful Patient," *New England Journal of Medicine* 298, no. 16 (April 1978): 883–87.

19   **"Heartsink" patients**   Shahady, "Difficult Patients."

19   **Patients who come in**   Scott Haig, "When the Patient Is a Googler," *Time,* November 8, 2007.

20   **"I groan when"**   Danielle Ofri, "Torment," *New England Journal of Medicine* 350, no. 22 (May 2004): 2233–36.

20 **"Mary" reached Dr. Levinson** Wendy Levinson, "Reflections: Mining for Gold," *Journal of General Internal Medicine* 8, no. 3 (March 1993): 172.

21 **when she hated Mary** Wendy Levinson to author, October 8, 2008.

22 **when a man walks** "Women and Heart Disease Facts," Women's Heart Foundation, www.womensheart.org.

22 **when she was a medical student** Nancy Snyderman, *Medical Myths That Can Kill You* (New York: Crown Publishers, 2008), 73.

23 **"To this day"** Snyderman, *Medical Myths That Can Kill You,* 81.

23 **set up a sneaky experiment** Cornelia M. Borkhoff et al., "The Effect of Patients' Sex on Physicians' Recommendations for Total Knee Arthroplasty," *Canadian Medical Association Journal* 178, no. 6 (March 11, 2008): 681–87.

24 **"Gender bias may"** Borkhoff, "The Effect of Patients' Sex on Physicians' Recommendations for Total Knee Arthroplasty," 681.

24 **They're less likely to receive kidney transplants** Borkhoff, "The Effect of Patients' Sex on Physicians' Recommendations for Total Knee Arthroplasty," 681.

24 **Women are also less likely** Arlene S. Bierman, "Sex Matters: Gender Disparities in Quality and Outcomes of Care," *Canadian Medical Association Journal* 177, no. 12 (December 2007): 1520.

24 **"some physicians take women's symptoms"** Borkhoff, *"The Effect of Patients' Sex on Physicians' Recommendations for Total Knee Arthroplasty,"* 684.

24 **black patients at Veterans Affairs hospitals** Jeff Whittle et al., "Racial Differences in the Use of Invasive Cardiovascular Procedures in the Department of Veterans Affairs Medical System," *New England Journal of Medicine,* vol. 329 (August 26, 1993): 621–27.

24–25 **African-American patients were less likely** Alan Zaslavsky and John Ayanian, "Integrating Research on Racial and Ethnic Disparities in Health Care Over Place and Time," *Medical Care* 43, no. 4 (April 2005): 303–7.

25 **black and Hispanic women** Nina A. Bickell, "Missed Opportunities: Racial Disparities in Adjuvant Breast Cancer Treatment," *Journal of Clinical Oncology* 24, no. 9 (March 2006): 1357–62. Jennifer Griggs, "Social and Racial Differences in Selection of Breast Cancer Adjuvant Chemotherapy Regimens," *Journal of Clinical Oncology* 25, no. 18 (June 2007): 2522–27. Griggs, "Racial Disparity in the Dose and Dose Intensity of Breast Cancer Adjuvant Chemotherapy," *Breast Cancer Research and Treatment* 81 (March 2003): 21–31.

25 **black women with breast cancer** Jean Yoon, "Symptom Management After Breast Cancer Treatment: Is It Influenced by Patient Characteristics?" *Breast Cancer Research and Treatment* 108, no. 1 (March 2008): 69–77.

25 **white patients were more likely** Joshua Tamayo-Sarver, "Racial and Ethnic Disparities in Emergency Department Analgesic Prescription," *American Journal of Public Health* 93, no. 12 (December 2003): 2067–73.

25 **researchers wrote a vignette** Alexander Green et al., "Implicit Bias

Among Physicians and Its Prediction of Thrombolysis Decisions for Black and White Patients," *Journal of General Internal Medicine* 22, no. 9 (July 2007): 1231–38.

25 **in one survey** Melanie Jay et al., "Physicians' Attitudes About Obesity and Their Associations with Competency and Specialty: A Cross-Sectional Study," *BMC Health Services Research* 9, no. 106 (June 2009).

26 **researchers at Rice University** M. R. Hebl and J. Xu, "Weighing the Care: Physicians' Reactions to the Size of a Patient," *International Journal of Obesity,* 25, no. 8 (August 2001): 1,246–52.

26 **medical students were more likely** Rebecca Puhl and Kelly D. Brownell, "Bias, Discrimination, and Obesity," *Obesity Research* 9, no. 12 (December 2001): 792.

26 **out of dozens of different categories** Puhl, "Bias, Discrimination, and Obesity," 792.

26 **48 percent of nurses** Puhl, "Bias, Discrimination, and Obesity," 792.

26 **24 percent said they were** Marlene B. Schwartz, "Weight Bias Among Health Professionals Specializing in Obesity," *Obesity Research* 11, no. 9 (September 2003): 1033–39.

28 **"Just as you would"** Elizabeth Cohen, "Five Ways to Find Dr. Right," www.cnn.com/empoweredpatient, February 14, 2008.

28 **once had a doctor** Christine Miserandino to author, November 19, 2008.

29 **pay close attention** John Santa to author, October 6, 2008.

31 **"There are lots of nice people"** Cohen, "Five Ways to Find Dr. Right."

33 **Dr. Joan Harrold** Elizabeth Cohen, "What to Expect from Your Doctor," www.cnn.com/empoweredpatient, February 28, 2008.

33 **if you're sick** Elizabeth Cohen, "What to Expect from Your Doctor," www.cnn.com/empoweredpatient, February 28, 2008.

34 **"Since when did"** Cohen, "Know When It's Time to Fire Your Doctor," www.cnn.com/empoweredpatient, August 16, 2007.

34 **"She told him she'd taken"** Cohen, "Know When It's Time to Fire Your Doctor."

34 **"Patients should have"** Cohen, "What to Expect from Your Doctor."

35 **"A lovely gentleman"** Cohen, "What to Expect from Your Doctor."

35 **Amy didn't have to** Cohen, "Five Ways to Find Dr. Right."

36 **"For example"** Howard Beckman to author, August 21, 2008.

37 **"He's just not that into you"** Julie Rottenberg and Elisa Zuritsky, "Pick-A-Little, Talk-A-Little," *Sex and the City,* HBO, season 6, episode 78 (original aired July 13, 2003).

38 **"If a doctor connects"** Wendy Levinson to author.

Chapter 3: Don't Leave a Doctor's Appointment Saying "Huh?"

41 **Most of us love** Paul Konowitz to author, December 17, 2008.

42 **"During my dermatology rotation"** Paul Konowitz, "The Last Patient of the Day," www.healthangle.com.

43 **Eighteen minutes** Larry B. Mauksch, "Relationship, Communication, and Efficiency in the Medical Encounter," *Archives of Internal Medicine* 168, no. 13 (July 2008): 1387–95.

44 **Now, about twenty-three** M. Kim Marvel, "Soliciting the Patient's Agenda: Have We Improved?" *Journal of the American Medical Association* 281, no. 3 (January 1999): 283–87.

44 **"The doctor blames"** Howard Beckman to author, August 21, 2008.

45 **On average, the patients asked** Sherrie Kaplan to author, August 4, 2009.

45 **"Most of us go"** Kaplan to author.

46 **A study of diabetics** Sheldon Greenfield et al., "Patients' Participation in Medical Care: Effects on Blood Sugar Control and Quality of Life in Diabetes, *Journal of General Internal Medicine* 3 (September–October 1988): 448–57.

46 **"What I really want"** Elizabeth Cohen, "Five Ways to Help Your Doctor Help You," www.cnn.com/empoweredpatient, April 3, 2008.

47 **"It's surprising"** Cohen, "Five Ways to Help Your Doctor Help You."

47 **"Don't count on"** Konowitz to author.

50 **First, ask yourself what symptoms** Cohen, "Five Ways to Help Your Doctor Help You."

51 **"Let them feel"** Konowitz to author.

51 **"Be polite but"** Elizabeth Cohen, "Sick? Doctor's Busy? Here's Help," www.cnn.com/empoweredpatient, December 9, 2008.

51 **She actually called** Cohen, "Sick? Doctor's Busy? Here's Help."

52 **"This is a true story"** Cohen, "Sick? Doctor's Busy? Here's Help."

53 **A Las Vegas man** Elizabeth Cohen, "Waiting for the Doctor . . . and Waiting and Waiting," www.cnn.com/empoweredpatient, October 23, 2008.

53 **He suggests** Cohen, "Waiting for the Doctor."

53 **"After fifteen minutes"** Cohen, "Waiting for the Doctor."

53 **"I ended up"** Cohen, "Waiting for the Doctor."

54 **"If a physician jumps"** Larry Mauksch to author, August 13, 2009.

55–56 **"They want to get patients"** Deepak Chopra to author, July 14, 2009.

56 **"If some aspect"** Mauksch to author, August 13, 2009.

Chapter 4: How to Avoid a Misdiagnosis

59 **Imagine waking up one day** Trisha Torrey, *You Bet Your Life! The 10 Mistakes Every Patient Makes (How to Fix Them to Get the Health Care You Deserve)* (Minneapolis: Langdon Street Press, 2010), 1–3. Trisha Torrey, "Trisha's Misdiagnosis Story," www.trishatorrey.com. Elizabeth Cohen, "Has Your Illness Been Misdiagnosed?" www.cnn.com/empoweredpatient, September 19, 2007.

59 **"What I learned"** Torrey, "Trisha's Misdiagnosis Story."

59 **"You have no choice"** Torrey, *You Bet Your Life!*

60 **the average survival time**   Irene M. Ghobrial et al., "Clinical Outcome of Patients with Subcutaneous Panniculitis-like T-Cell Lymphoma," *Leukemia and Lymphoma* 46, no. 5 (May 2005): 703–8.

61 **Lymos that originate in the brain**   Sakeer Hussain et al., "Primary Intracranial Leiomyosarcoma: Report of a Case and Review of the Literature," *Sarcoma* 2006 (December 2006): 1–3.

62 **the most common malignant brain tumor**   American Cancer Society, "Detailed Guide: Brain/CNS Tumors in Adults," cancer.org, November 12, 2009.

62 **several studies**   Mark L. Graber, "Diagnostic Error in Internal Medicine," *Archives of Internal Medicine* 31, no. 2 (February 2005): 1493–99.

62 **as high as**   Gordon D. Schiff et al., "Diagnosing Diagnosis Errors: Lessons from a Multi-Institutional Collaborative Project in Advances in Patient Safety." *From Research to Implementation* 2: Concepts and Methodology, U.S. Agency for Healthcare Research and Quality, ahrg.gov, February 2005, 255–78.

63 **pathologist made the wrong call**   Stephen S. Raab et al., "Clinical Impact and Frequency of Anatomic Pathology," *Cancer* 104, issue 10 (October 10, 2005): 2205–13.

63 **they disagreed**   E. Potchen, "Measuring Observer Performance in Chest Radiology: Some Experiences," *Journal of the American College of Radiology* 3, no. 6 (2000): 423–32. Jerome Groopman, *How Doctors Think* (New York: Houghton Mifflin, 2007), 179.

63 **learned from infectious-disease experts**   Andrew Pavia to author, November 24, 2009.

64 *966 testing-process errors*   J. Hickner, "Testing Process Errors and Their Harms and Consequences Reported from Family Medicine Practices: A study of the American Academy of Family Physicians National Research Network," *Quality and Safety in Health Care* 17 (2008): 194–200.

64 **"A doctor's office is always"**   Robert Lamberts, "Getting Along: Part 2—Patient Rules," www.distractible.org, August 11, 2008.

65 **"Diagnostic errors are simply not"**   Mark L. Graber, "Diagnostic Errors in Medicine: A Case of Neglect," *Journal on Quality and Patient Safety* 31, no. 2 (February 2005): 108.

65 **"Diagnosing is the most important thing"**   Pat Croskerry to author, January 21, 2009.

65 **When Doug Smith**   Elizabeth Cohen, "Your Private Health Details May Already Be Online," www.cnn.com/empoweredpatient, June 5, 2008.

67 **"I told her to go"**   Cohen, "Is Grandma Drugged Up?" www.cnn.com/empoweredpatient, May 29, 2008.

67 **High School Girl Diagnoses Her Own Disease**   Elizabeth Cohen, *"Teen Diagnoses Her Own Disease in Science Class,"* www.cnn.com/empoweredpatient, June 11, 2009.

68 **"I learned . . . I should have symptoms"**   Torrey, *You Bet Your Life!* 2.

70 **"Most people aren't aware"**   Croskerry to author.

71 **"No news is not good news"**   Elizabeth Cohen, "Five Commonly Mis-diagnosed Diseases," www.cnn.com/empoweredpatient, October 3, 2007.

71 **made this question famous**   Groopman, *How Doctors Think*, 263.

72 **"Anchoring is a shortcut"**   Groopman, *How Doctors Think*, 65.

72 **several diseases could have been**   Corey Siegel to author, September 18, 2009.

74 **"When you say you're tired"**   Jerome Kassirer to author, January 14, 2009.

75 **Even something as simple**   Groopman, *How Doctors Think*, 158.

76 **a patient's diagnosis of tuberculosis**   Tejal K. Gandhi, "Fumbled Handoffs: One Dropped Ball After Another," *Annals of Internal Medicine* 142, no. 5 (March 2005): 352–58.

77 **a young woman who complained**   Cohen, "Has Your Illness Been Misdiagnosed?"

78 **"Properly educated"**   Mark L. Graber, Taking Steps Towards a Safer Future: Measures to Promote Timely and Accurate Medical Diagnosis, *American Journal of Medicine* 121, no. 5A (May 2008): S43–S46.

Chapter 5: How to Become an Internet MD (Medical Detective)

81 **"These resolutions"**   "AMA Suggests Resolutions for a Healthy New Year," press release, American Medical Association, December 26, 2001.

81 **"One [of my doctors] commented"**   Tom Ferguson and the E-Patient Scholars Working Group, "E-patients: How They Help Us Heal Health Care," www.epatients.net, 2007, 14.

82 **"went wild with fury"**   Ferguson, "E-patients," 14.

82 **"my child's GI [doctor]"**   Ferguson, "E-patients," 14.

82 **"I asked him"**   Tara Parker-Pope, "Lessons Learned from Doctors, Patients, and my Mother," *Wall Street Journal*, August 28, 2007.

83 **One morning in 1994**   Ferguson, "E-patients," 1.

84 **Sixteen-year-old Darrah Sandmaier**   Ferguson, "E-patients," 2. Marian Sandmaier, "Listening for Zebras: The Doctors Dismissed Her Daughter's Headaches as a Common Breed. Every Instinct Told Her They Were Wrong," *Washington Post*, June 3, 2003.

85 **Two doctors had now**   Ferguson, "E-patients," 3.

86 **When Dr. Kenneth Youner**   Kenneth Youner to author, March 8, 2009.

86 **"IL-2 is the only therapy"**   Detailed Guide: Kidney Cancer Biologic Therapy (Immunotherapy), American Cancer Society, www.cancer.org, last revised May 14, 2009.

87 **Fay Sutton learned of a treatment**   Dorothy Sutton to author, March 13, 2009. Jan Guthrie to author, February 18, 2009.

88 **38 percent believed**   Elizabeth Murray et al., "The Impact of Health Information on the Internet on Health Care and the Physician-Patient Relationship: National U.S. Survey among 1,050 U.S. Physicians," *Journal of Medical Internet Research* 5, no. 3 (August 2003).

88 **"hard time," "headache"** Farah Ahmad et al., "Are Physicians Ready for Patients with Internet-Based Health Information?" *Journal of Medical Internet Research* 8, no. 3 (September 2006).

89 **"Our patients are turning"** Paul C. Coelho, "The Internet: Increasing Information, Decreasing Certainty," *Journal of the American Medical Association* 280, no. 16 (October 1998): 1,454.

89 **"A little knowledge"** Richard J. Bold, "A Young Surgeon's Perspective," *Archives of Surgery* 140, no. 3 (March 2005): 254–57.

89 **"Most [patients] know it's annoying"** Ahmad, "Are Physicians Ready for Patients with Internet-Based Health Information?"

90 **You'll need to use your common sense** For more information on smart Internet surfing, see Elizabeth Cohen, "Tips for Savvy Medical Web Surfing," www.cnn.com/empoweredpatient, February 21, 2008.

91 **Two-thirds of all Internet health searchers** Susannah Fox, "Online Health Search 2006," Pew Internet & American Life Project, October 2006, 5.

92 **she found review articles** Cohen, "Tips for Savvy Medical Web Surfing."

93 **she owes her life** Elizabeth Cohen, "*The Life and Death of an Empowered Patient,*" www.cnn.com/empoweredpatient, February 26, 2009.

94 **We report two patients** Keyvan Nouri, "Imiquimod for the Treatment of Bowen's Disease and Invasive Squamous Cell Carcinoma," *Journal of Drugs in Dermatology* 2, no. 6 (December 2003): 669–73.

97 **"smart people write"** Elizabeth Cohen, "How to Get Kennedy-esque Health Care on Your Budget," www.cnn.com/empoweredpatient, August 27, 2009.

97 **"Stroke them a little"** Jan Guthrie to author, February 18, 2009.

97 **"She went to New York once"** Guthrie to author.

98 **go to the public-relations** Krista Kordt to author, May 25, 2009.

99 **"Plan in advance"** Elizabeth Cohen, "Are You a Cyberchondriac?" www.cnn.com/empoweredpatient, December 20, 2007.

99 **"I was studying"** Cohen, "Are You a Cyberchondriac?"

100 **"Understand that it is common"** Robert Lamberts to author, February 22, 2009.

101 **"Internet junkies"** John Castaldo, "Internet Use and the Doctor-Patient Relationship: The Good, the Bad, and the Ugly," *Neurology Today* 8, no. 13 (July 2008): 3–4.

101 **"Don't say"** Robert Lamberts to author, February 22, 2009.

101 **"Boil down your links"** Charles Smith to author, February 22, 2009.

102 **"Patients are bypassing"** Manjula Gunawardane, "My Patient on My-Space: E-patients and the Evolution of Healthcare on the Web," presentation at the University of Maryland, www.umm.edu, March 17, 2008.

102 **"Embracing the Internet"** Corey A. Siegel, "Embracing the Internet for Progress in Shared Decision-Making," *Inflammatory Bowel Disease* 13, no.12 (December 2007): 1579–80.

102 **"Welcome to the world"**   Hedy S. Wald et al., "Untangling the Web: The Impact of Internet Use on Health Care and the Physician-Patient Relationship," *Patient Education and Counseling* 68, no. 3 (November 2007): 218–24.

102 **"Accept the fact"**   Castaldo, "Internet Use and the Doctor-Patient Relationship."

102 **"I have a million things"**   Smith to author.

103 **"You will find"**   Castaldo, "Internet Use and the Doctor-Patient Relationship."

Chapter 6: You vs. the Insurance Industry

106 **Patsy Bates was cutting**   CNN transcript, "Anderson Cooper 360," February 22, 2009.

108 **She initially thought**   Elizabeth Cohen, "Don't Get Scammed by Fake Health Plans," www.cnn.com/empoweredpatient, June 3, 2009.

109 **"Medical discount cards"**   Cohen, "Don't Get Scammed by Fake Health Plans."

109 **Between 2000 and 2002**   Cohen, "Don't Get Scammed by Fake Health Plans."

110 **The National Association of Insurance Commissioners**   Cohen, "Don't Get Scammed by Fake Health Plans."

110 **"Will the company"**   Elizabeth Cohen, "How to Shop for Health Insurance," www.cnn.com/empoweredpatient, March 12, 2009.

112 **Karen Tumulty, a *Time* magazine writer**   "The Health-Care Crisis Hits Home," *Time,* March 5, 2009.

112 **"It's never, never"**   Nancy Metcalf to author, November 6, 2009.

113 **Generally speaking, HMOs**   "The Managed Care Answer Guide," Patient Advocate Foundation, www.patientadvocate.org.

115 **some policies have**   Nancy Davenport-Ennis to author, November 4, 2009.

116 **Bailey died**   Elizabeth Cohen, "Tips to Effectively Battle Your Insurance Company," www.cnn.com/empoweredpatient, July 20, 2007.

118 **"You may go through"**   Cohen, "Tips to Effectively Battle Your Insurance Company."

118 **"When they saw"**   Cohen, "Tips to Effectively Battle Your Insurance Company."

Chapter 7: How to Get Good Drugs Cheap

121 **More than $100**   All prices are from www.crbestbuydrugs.org, accessed March 12, 2009.

121 **Ninety-one percent of seniors**   Allison Woo et al., "Prescription Drug Costs: Background Brief," the Henry J. Kaiser Family Foundation. Updated February 2010, www.kaiseredu.org.

121 **Prices for widely used** "Looking to Save on Drugs? Go Generic," American Association of Retired Persons (AARP), April 16, 2009.

122 **paying $102 a month** Consumer Reports Best Buy Drugs, crbestbuy drugs.org.

122 **helped more than 44,000 people** Nancy Davenport-Ennis et al, "Patient Advocate Foundation: Patient Data Analysis Report for 2007," eleventh edition, available at www.copays.org.

122 **higher-income adults** Laurie E. Felland and James D. Reschovsky, "More Non Elderly Americans Face Problems Affording Prescription Drugs," Tracking Report No. 22, Center for Studying Health System Change, January 2009, available at www.hschange.com.

125 **"She should call"** Jennifer Niebyl to author, March 17, 2009.

125 **"Most providers** Diane Ashton to author, March 16, 2009.

126 **"We have no idea"** Elizabeth Cohen, "Ten 'Secrets' You Shouldn't Keep from Your Doctor," www.cnn.com/empoweredpatient, March 5, 2009.

126 **Dr. Adair said** "Should You Really Take Those Drug Samples?" www.cnn.com/empoweredpatient, April 24, 2008.

126 **"Samples look like they're free"** Cohen, "Should You Really Take Those Drug Samples?"

127 **Consumer Reports has a guide** "Shopper's Guide to Prescription Drugs Number 5—Assistance Programs," www.consumerreports.org, 2007.

127 **Consumer Reports also offers tips** "Shopper's Guide to Prescription Drugs Number 1—Pill Splitting," www.consumerreports.org, 2006.

Chapter 8: Don't Fall for Medical Marketing

132 **Linda Lewis learned the hard way** Elizabeth Cohen, "Don't Become a Victim of Medical Marketing," www.cnn.com/empoweredpatient, August 21, 2008.

132 **her surgeon had accepted** Cohen, "Don't Become a Victim of Medical Marketing."

132 **$8 million two other physicians received** Cohen, "Don't Become a Victim of Medical Marketing."

133 **"He told us there was no hope"** Dina Foster to author, March 28, 2009.

133 **"At no time was Interleukin"** Dina Foster to author.

134 **"I think the real failing"** James Yang to author, March 10, 2009.

134 **"If a doctor's taking money"** Dina Foster to author.

134 **"begin in medical school"** David Blumenthal, "Doctors and Drug Companies," *New England Journal of Medicine* 351, no. 18 (October 2004): 1885–90.

134 **In a 2007 study** Eric G. Campbell et al., "A National Survey of Physician-Industry Relationships," *New England Journal of Medicine* 356, no. 17 (April 2007).

134 **the average doctor meets**   Kenneth V. Iserson, "Politely Refuse the Pen and Note Pad: Gifts from Industry to Physicians Harm Patients," *Annals of Thoracic Surgery* 84, Issue 4 (October 2007): 1077–84.

134 **in 2007 Americans spent $287 million**   Elizabeth Cohen, "Ten Ways to Save on Prescription Drugs," www.cnn.com/empoweredpatient, March 19, 2009.

134 **"a battle is being waged"**   Iserson, "Politely Refuse the Pen and Note Pad."

135 **when a doctor met with**   Ashley Wazana "Physicians and the Pharmaceutical Industry: Is a Gift Ever Just a Gift?" *Journal of the American Medical Association* 283, no. 3 (January 2000): 373–80.

135 **A financial analysis . . . at Yale University**   Dick Wittink, "Analysis of ROI for Pharmaceutical Promotion," www.rxpromoroi.org, September 18, 2002.

135 **they spend $12 billion a year**   L. Lewis Wall and Douglas Brown, "The High Cost of Free Lunch," *Obstetrics and Gynecology* 110, no. 1 (July 2007): 169–73. Iserson, "Politely Refuse the Pen and Note Pad."

135 **"otherwise, why would the pharmaceutical industry"**   Mark W. Mahowald and Michel Cramer Bornemann, "What? Influenced by Industry? Not Me!" *Sleep Medicine* 6 (2005), 389–90.

135 **"The industry only does things"**   Kathleen Slattery-Moschkau to author, March 27, 2009.

136 **"circling the day"**   Jamie Reidy to author, March 27, 2009.

137 **"My research found"**   Jamie Reidy, *Hard Sell: The Evolution of a Viagra Salesman* (Kansas City: Andrews McMeel, 2005), 75.

137 **"Our training in sales school"**   Shahram Ahari to author, March 28, 2009.

138 **"He just said it in passing"**   Jamie Reidy to author.

138 **"His numbers went through the roof!"**   Jamie Reidy to author.

138 **the Food and Drug Administration**   "Questions and Answers on Trovafloxacin Public Health Advisory," U.S. Food and Drug Administration, 1999.

139 **None of the 7,000 patients**   FDA, "Questions and Answers on Trovafloxacin Public Health Advisory," www.fda.gov, updated April 30, 2009.

139 **Doctors at the Mayo Clinic discovered**   "Questions and Answers About Withdrawal of Fenfluramine (Pondimin) and Dexfenfluramine (Redux)," September 18, 1997, updated July 7, 2005, ,www.fda.gov.

139 **Then there's the antibiotic Raxar**   "New, Improved and Dangerous," www.smartmoney.com, February 22, 2001.

139 **Merck pulled Vioxx**   "Vioxx (Rofecoxib) Questions and Answers," updated June 18, 2009.

140 **"I was part of Lilly's elite"**   Ahari to author.

140 **"Every day"**   Reidy to author.

141 **"I'd call my mom and dad"**   Gene Carbona to author, April 2, 2009.

141 **"I left the industry"** Slattery-Moschkau to author.

141 **"I looked at it"** Carbona to author.

142 **the drug industry decided to police** "Code on Interactions with Healthcare Professionals," Pharmaceutical Research and Manufacturers of America, revised July 2008.

143 **"If you see an extremely attractive"** Cohen, "Don't Become a Victim of Medical Marketing."

143 **they're still allowed** "Code on Interactions with Healthcare Professionals," Pharmaceutical Research and Manufacturers of America.

144 **This psychiatrist was removed** Gayle White and Craig Schneider, "Depression Expert at Emory Pulls out of Research," *Atlanta Journal Constitution,* October 14, 2008. Craig Schneider, "Controversial Emory Researcher Leaving," *Atlanta Journal Constitution,* October 30, 2009.

145 **Much of the money came from Wyeth Pharmaceuticals** Gayle White and Craig Schneider, "Depression Expert at Emory Pulls out of Research," *Atlanta Journal Constitution,* October 14, 2008.

146 **the rules have changed** "Code on Interactions with Healthcare Professionals," Pharmaceutical Research and Manufacturers of America.

146 **"U2 is coming to town"** Carbona to author.

146 **They can still pay for doctors' meals** "Code on Interactions with Healthcare Professionals," Pharmaceutical Research and Manufacturers of America.

146 **"Let's say your investment counselor"** Cohen, "Don't Become a Victim of Medical Marketing."

Chapter 9: Don't Let a Hospital Kill You

149 **He says he's alive today** Elizabeth Cohen, "Picking the Right Hospital Can Save Your Life," www.cnn.com/empoweredpatient, July 26, 2007.

149 **can significantly reverse** "Most U.S. Hospitals Don't Provide Powerful Acute Stroke Drug to Medicare Patients," American Heart Association, February 19, 2009.

150 **"the shortest fifteen minutes of my life"** Cohen, "Picking the Right Hospital Can Save Your Life."

150 **actor Dennis Quaid** Dennis Quaid to author, April 21, 2009.

152 **An investigation by Cedars-Sinai** "Statement of Michael L. Langberg, MD, Chief Medical Officer, Cedars-Sinai Medical Center," press release from Cedars-Sinai Medical Center, November 20, 2007.

153 **in 2006, three infants died** "Actor tells House panel of newborn twins' overdose," www.cnn.com, May 14, 2008.

153 **In 2008, fourteen infants** "Second Twin Dies as Hospital Probes Heparin Overdoses," www.cnn.com, July 10, 2008.

153 **Cedars-Sinai switched to saline** Press release, Cedars-Sinai Medical Center, December 4, 2007.

153 **"The first overdose occurred"** Quaid to author.

153 **Dennis Quaid's Tips** Quaid to author and Frank Federico, "The Five Rights of Medication Administration," Institute for Healthcare Improvement, July 11, 2007.

154 **"We were lucky"** Quaid to author.

154 **98,000 people die** Linda T. Kohn et al., eds., *To Err Is Human: Building a Safer Health System* (Washington, DC: National Academy Press, 1999). Available at www.iom.edu.

154 **at least one medication error** Philip Aspden et al. *Preventing Medication Errors: Quality Chasm Series* (Washington, DC: National Academies Press, 2007). Available at www.iom.edu.

154 **"It's like a major airline crash"** Quaid to author.

154 **"If it can happen"** "Dennis Quaid Recounts Twins' Drug Ordeal," *60 Minutes,* CBS News, August 24, 2008.

155 **99,000 Americans die each year** "Estimates of Healthcare-Associated Infections," U.S. Centers for Disease Control and Prevention, modified June 15, 2009.

155 **one out of every twenty-two patients** David S. Martin, "Unsung Heroes Work Hard to Cut Hospital-Acquired Infections," www.cnn.com/empoweredpatient, July 9, 2009.

155 **with only 40 percent adhering** John M. Boyce and Didier Pittet, "Guideline for Hand Hygiene in Health-Care Settings: Recommendations of the Healthcare Infection Control Practices Advisory Committee and the HICPAC/SHEA/APIC/IDSA Hand Hygiene Task Force," *Morbidity and Mortality Weekly Report,* U.S. Centers for Disease Control and Prevention 51 (RR16), www.cdc.gov (October 25, 2002), 1–44.

155 **Edith Rodriguez lay on the floor** Charles Ornstein, "Tale of Last 90 Minutes of Woman's Life," *Los Angeles Times,* May 20, 2007.

155 **Rodriguez died in the ER** Charles Ornstein, "How a Hospital Death Became a Cause Célèbre," *Los Angeles Times,* June 15, 2007.

155 **the average total waiting time** Elizabeth Cohen, "Five Things Not to Do in the ER," www.cnn.com/empoweredpatient, January 17, 2008.

155 **one in four heart-attack patients** Cohen, "Five Things Not to Do in the ER."

155 **"Ridiculously long wait times"** Cohen, "Five Things Not to Do in the ER."

156 **heart-attack patients have a higher chance** Cohen, "Picking the Right Hospital Can Save Your Life."

156 **very low-birthweight babies** Cohen, "Picking the Right Hospital Can Save Your Life."

156 **"A lot of people think"** Cohen, "Picking the Right Hospital Can Save Your Life."

157 **"If we're going to spend hours on the Internet"** Cohen, "Picking the Right Hospital Can Save Your Life."

158 **"Let's say I'm having a surgery"** Cohen, "Picking the Right Hospital Can Save Your Life."

158 **"They'll talk to me professionally"** Cohen, "Five Things Not to Do in the ER."

158 **"There's a myth out there"** Cohen, "Five Things Not to Do in the ER."

159 **"Speak up"** Cohen, "Five Things Not to Do in the ER."

159 **"Even the smallest hospitals"** Cohen, "Five Things Not to Do in the ER."

159 **"I personally saw a mom"** Elizabeth Cohen, "Five Ways to Avoid Medication Mistakes," www.cnn.com/empoweredpatient, November 29, 2007.

160 **"Had I not been there to intercept"** Cohen, "Five Ways to Avoid Medication Mistakes."

162 **Josh Nahum loved a thrill** Elizabeth Cohen, "Don't Let a Hospital Kill You," www.cnn.com/empoweredpatient, May 1, 2008.

162 **"One nurse"** Cohen, "Don't Let a Hospital Kill You."

163 **heat up your car** Cohen, "Don't Let a Hospital Kill You."

163 **"If the patient is awake"** Cohen, "Don't Let a Hospital Kill You."

163 **A central line is inserted** "Patient Information Series—Central Venous Catheter," American Thoracic Society, www.thoracic.org.

164 **250,000 people** "Ending Health Care–Associated Infections," Agency for Healthcare Research and Quality, U.S. Department of Health and Human Services, www.ahrq.gov, October 2009.

164 **"My brother was in the hospital"** Cohen, "Don't Let a Hospital Kill You."

164 **"I didn't see you"** Cohen, "Don't Let a Hospital Kill You."

164 **"In the hospital"** Cohen, "Don't Let a Hospital Kill You."

Epilogue

173 **Gilles pointed out** Gilles Frydman to author, December 7, 2009.

173 **"You have brains"** Theodor Seuss Geisel, *Oh, the Places You'll Go* (New York: Random House, 1990), 2.

Appendix

186 **It took the Trim family** Elizabeth Cohen, "Five Mistakes That Will Land You in Medical Debt," www.cnn.com/empoweredpatient, August 28, 2008.

186 **A 2008 report** Cohen, "Five Mistakes That Will Land You in Medical Debt."

186 **72 million Americans** Sara R. Collins et al., "Losing Ground: How the Loss of Adequate Health Insurance Is Burdening Working Families—Findings from the Commonwealth Fund Biennial Health Insurance Surveys, 2001–2007," Commonwealth Fund, August 20, 2008.

186 **Nearly one-third** Mark Rukavina, "The Financial Burden of Health Care," *Communities and Banking,* Federal Reserve Bank of Boston (Summer 2009), 10.

186 **nearly one out of every four Americans** Elizabeth Cohen, "Tips to Effectively Battle Your Insurance Company."

186 **"Two-thirds of the people"** Cohen, "Five Mistakes That Will Land You in Medical Debt."

186 **"When medical debt hits"** Cohen, "Five Mistakes That Will Land You in Medical Debt."

187 **"The most dangerous thing"** Cohen, "Five Mistakes That Will Land You in Medical Debt."

187 **"I had a client once"** Cohen, "Five Mistakes That Will Land You in Medical Debt."

187 **"People think they have to pay** Elizabeth Cohen, "Five Mistakes That Will Land You in Medical Debt."

187 *My Healthcare Is Killing Me* The entire book can be downloaded for free at www.myhealthcareiskillingme.com.

188 **visit the website of Medical Billing Advocates of America** The website for Medical Billing Advocates of America is www.billadvocates .com. The website for the Fairness Foundation is www.fairnessfoundation .org. The website for the National Foundation for Credit Counseling is www.nfcc.org. The website for the Patient Advocate Foundation is www .patientadvocate.org.

190 **I asked four ER doctors** Cohen, "How to Get Help in a Hurry in the ER," www.cnn.com/empoweredpatient, June 25, 2009.

Index

About the Author

ELIZABETH COHEN is senior medical correspondent for CNN and author of the popular "Empowered Patient" column on cnn.com. She received her master's degree in public health from Boston University and her bachelor's degree from Columbia University in New York City. She lives in Atlanta, Georgia, with her husband, Tal Cohen, and their four daughters.